ILLUSTRATED CASE HISTORIES

 Mosby-Wolfe

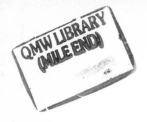

Project Manager:	Jane Hurd-Cosgrave
Developmental Editor:	Jennifer Prast
Production:	Jane Tozer
Index:	Anita Reid
Cover design:	Lara Last
Publisher:	Richard Furn

Copyright © 1995 Times Mirror International Publishers Limited.

Published in 1995 by Mosby-Wolfe, an imprint of Times Mirror International Publishers Limited.

Originated by Mandarin Offset, Ltd., Hong Kong.

Printed by Grafos S. A. Arte sobre papel, Barcelona, Spain.

ISBN 0 7234 2146 3

For full details of all Times Mirror International Publishers Limited titles, please write to Times Mirror International Publishers Limited, Lynton House, 7–12 Tavistock Square, London WC1H 9LB, England.

A CIP catalogue record for this book is available from the British Library.

Library of Congress Cataloging-in-Publication Data has been applied for.

Contents

PREFACE

This book sets out a series of case histories of patients seen over the last two or three years. The cases encompass a wide range of different chest conditions, and we have not hesitated to involve our colleagues when we needed their expertise. This book is, however, not intended to cover the whole of chest medicine. Our main aim has been to provide illustrative cases which require thought in the diagnosis, and to give an insight to the current management of a wide range of chest problems.

The format of these cases is one of question and answer and, wherever possible, we have placed the answers on a separate page. Each of the cases is self-contained, and it is intended that they can be read in any order that suits the reader. We have designed the book to help post graduates who are involved in higher examinations. However, we hope that the case reports are of use to any qualified doctor and to more senior medical students.

It is quite likely that some points, particularly those involving patient management, may be challenged by our readers. However, any such disagreement should stimulate the reader to go to the standard textbooks, specialist monographs, journals and national guidelines (e.g. those for asthma and pneumonia).

We hope readers will enjoy using this book of illustrated case histories, and that it is found to be a useful teaching exercise.

ACKNOWLEDGEMENTS

First, we would like to thank our colleagues who provided five of the case histories: Dr. Peter Davies, known for his expert knowledge of mycobacterial diseases, contributed three illustrative cases of tuberculosis; Dr. Martin Walshaw, who runs the specialised adult cystic fibrosis service for Merseyside, reported one of his patients; our senior registrar, Dr. David Spence, wrote and illustrated the two cases of breathing disorders during sleep.

Collecting the illustrations has involved many individuals. We would like to acknowledge Mr. Richard Hancock of our Medical Illustration Department for his assistance and illustrations. We would particularly like to thank Dr. Bill Taylor, who has painstakingly provided all the pathology slides, and Dr. Joe Danher for his help with the radiographic illustrations. Dr Nick Beeching, who has written a sister volume on infectious diseases, was instrumental in encouraging us to undertake this work, and gave us much valuable advice. We also thank Dr Peter Calverley, Dr Gary Jamieson, Dr John Littler, Mr Ajab Soorae, Dr. Robert Thompson, Dr. Charles Van Heyningen, Dr. Tony Morris and Dr. John Cheeseborough. We apologise if we have inadvertently omitted any other names from the list of acknowledgements.

We are grateful to our publishers, particularly Jennifer Prast, whose encouragement and gentle persuasion has enabled us to complete the work. We also thank Jane Hurd-Cosgrave and other members of the publishing team for their help and understanding.

Finally, writing such a work is yet another impingement on family life, and we would both like to thank our families for their whole-hearted support and encouragement.

Case 1
Breathlessness and an abnormal chest radiograph

A man of 44 years presented with worsening breathlessness. He had been perfectly well in his youth and indeed until about six years before. He had played semi-professional football until he was 30, and had performed a heavy job as a steel erector until three years earlier when it became clear that he was unable to keep up with his workmates and the workteam were not getting their bonuses. Since then the breathlessness had worsened, so that although he could still walk half a mile at his own pace, he was unable to cope with gardening or handyman jobs any more. He did not have a cough and had had no phlegm since stopping smoking seven years earlier. There was no family history of chest disease and no history of atopy or allergy. He was not taking medication, and drank alcohol only occasionally. On examination, he was pink with no finger clubbing, but he was breathless while undressing. He had no abnormal cardiovascular signs, and in the chest no signs were noted except that the breath sounds seemed distant and the percussion note mildly reduced all over. However, the chest radiograph was clearly abnormal (**1**), and this finding was confirmed on a computed tomography (CT) scan (**2**). A Rotex needle biopsy of the pleura was performed (**3**) from which the diagnosis was made. **4** is a larger biopsy from a similar case. His lung function tests were abnormal (*see* **Investigations**).

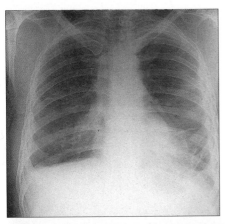

1 Posterior-anterior (PA) chest radiograph.

2 CT scan of the mid chest.

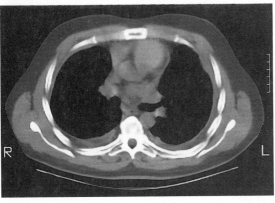

Case 1

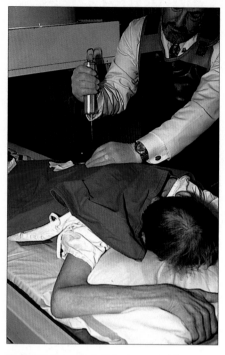

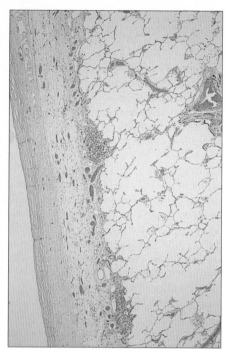

3 Rotex needle being inserted into chest.

4 Pleural biopsy.

Investigations

	Actual	Predicted
Forced expiratory volume in one second (FEV$_1$):	1.2 L	3.3 L
FEV$_1$ post-salbutamol:	1.3 L	
Forced vital capacity (FVC):	1.5 L	4.2 L
Residual volume (RV) (helium dilution):	1.1 L	2.2 L
Total lung capacity (TLC):	2.65 L	6.4 L
Diffusing capacity (D$_L$co):	5.3 ml/min/mmHg	8.2 ml/min/mmHg

QUESTIONS

1. What process is going on to produce these findings?
2. What are the possible causes and what extra history would you elicit?
3. What is the likely prognosis, and what treatment would you consider?
4. Should this man see a solicitor?

ANSWERS

1. The plain PA chest radiograph shows that there is a dense thickening of the pleura around both lungs. The pleura is visible as a white layer up to 12 mm thick lining the inside of the ribs. An important feature which indicates that this is diffuse pleural thickening rather than pleural plaques is the involvement and obliteration of the costophrenic angle. The CT scan shows this in cross-section, and also demonstrates how the pleura is encasing and restricting the underlying lung, resulting in the severe restrictive impairment apparent on the lung function tests. The pleural biopsy shows that the pleura is composed of fibrous tissue and that there is no evidence of malignancy.

2. There are a number of recognised causes of diffuse pleural thickening. Asbestos exposure is probably the commonest, with the pleural disease developing often years after the exposure and sometimes progressing in a step-wise manner. After specific questioning, this man admitted to having spent his early years as an apprentice in the ship repair industry, where he had stripped asbestos from old boilers and piping on a regular basis for about six years with no respiratory protection at all. Thereafter he had moved into the building industry, where he had no known further contact with asbestos. The progressive history, clinical picture and biopsy are all consistent with this explanation, although proof is impossible in real life.

   Connective tissue disorders can cause pleural fibrosis. Systemic lupus erythematosus (SLE) can cause a shrinking pleuritis with a restrictive picture, similar to this but often without obvious radiological abnormality. Rheumatoid disease results in effusions that usually resolve spontaneously and do not cause marked restriction or radiological abnormality. This man's rheumatoid factor and antinuclear factor were both negative, and his erythrocyte sedimentation rate (ESR) was normal. Most importantly, there were no other signs or symptoms in other systems to support a diagnosis of connective tissue disorder.

   Third, drugs such as practolol (a beta-blocking drug withdrawn in the 1970s) and methysergide (used for migraine) can produce precisely this clinical picture. Even on careful questioning, no such drug history could be obtained.

   On balance, therefore, asbestos is the most likely cause. Confirmation of asbestos exposure may be available later from postmortem tissue, in which the asbestos fibre count (**5**) may be markedly elevated and asbestos bodies may be visible (**6**).

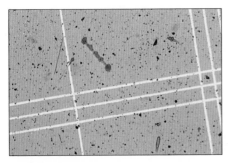

5 Asbestos fibres from a dried lung specimen in a counting chamber.

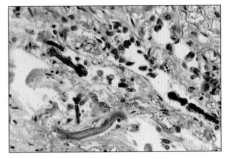

6 Asbestos bodies in the lung tissue.

Case 1

3. The prognosis of asbestos-related diffuse pleural thickening is very variable. If there is no further exposure, some cases may remain stable for many years, whereas others can show a step-wise progression with deterioration every few years, or may seem to progress relentlessly. The prognosis in this man is likely to be slow, but given his already severely impaired lung function, it is probable that over the next decade or so his activities will become more restricted with the prospect of respiratory failure and premature death. There is no specific therapy known to alter the progression of pleural fibrosis, but some surgeons would consider trying pleurectomy as they would for unilateral pleural thickening secondary to empyema. This man was offered surgical help but declined.

4. Asbestos exposure can cause a variety of respiratory problems, which may or may not justify a legal claim. The following list describes the range of pathology that can result from asbestos exposure.

   a. Despite media and pressure-group publicity, exposure to asbestos does not equate with disease or disability, and therefore no claims may be made for exposure alone.
   b. Simple pleural plaques, which are often calcified and which usually cause no symptoms (**7**).
   c. Benign pleural effusions, which are unilateral, yield straw-coloured uninfected fluid when aspirated, and resolve spontaneously (**8**).
   d. Diffuse bilateral pleural thickening (as here) (**9**).
   e. Asbestosis, which is defined as fibrosis of the lung tissue, and should not be confused with simple exposure alone or the other conditions in this list (**10**).
   f. Mesothelioma of the pleura (**11**) or peritoneum .
   g. Lung cancer of the right lower lobe (usually only accepted as asbestos-related when there is also proven asbestosis present) (**12**).

Anyone who develops conditions c to g above is likely to be judged to have a 'proscribed disease' and receive modest compensation under the UK government-run scheme. In addition, sufferers with conditions b to g may make a claim in the civil courts (for what are often larger amounts) against their former employers and/or their insurers. Choosing a specialist solicitor is important, and often the trade unions are a helpful advice source.

If this had been due to drugs there could also be a valid claim, but the outcome of such a claim is much less clear and more difficult to prove.

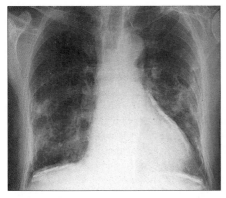

7 Chest radiograph showing simple pleural plaques.

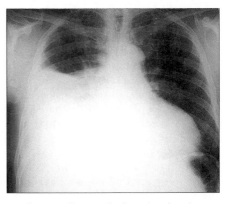

8 Chest radiograph showing benign pleural effusion.

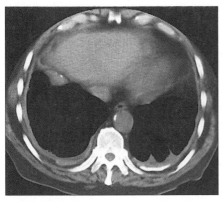

9 CT scan showing diffuse bilateral pleural thickening.

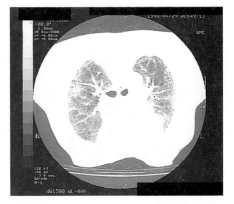

10 CT scan showing fibrosis of the lung tissue.

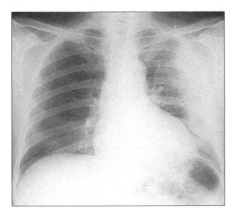

11 Chest radiograph showing mesothelioma of the pleura.

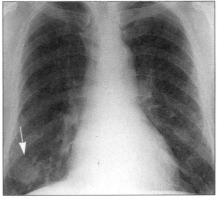

12 Chest radiograph showing a large white mass (*arrowed*) and asbestosis.

Case 2
The sleepy giant

A 52-year-old gentleman (1) presented to the accident and emergency department with a five-week history of increasing swelling of his legs and genitalia. He had a 20-year history of breathlessness, and for the previous two years had rarely managed to leave his first-floor flat. For the five weeks before admission he had been unable to get out of a chair, and had been sleeping most of the time. His past medical history included an operation for a 'hole in the heart' at the age of 12, and he had been told he had asthma but was on no regular medication for this. He had never smoked. He had difficulty keeping awake during the taking of the history, and on direct questioning admitted to falling asleep frequently during conversations. His wife said he snored heavily, and she had observed spells during which his breathing became quiet, terminated by a snort. On examination he was morbidly obese, weighing in excess of 150 kg. He was centrally cyanosed and had gross pitting oedema of his lower body. His jugular venous pressure (JVP) was elevated by 6 cm. Apart from shallow, rapid respirations and a left thoracotomy scar, examination of his respiratory system was unremarkable. Cardiovascular examination was normal, as was the abdomen apart from obesity and striae. Arterial blood gases are shown in the **Investigations**. He also had renal impairment.

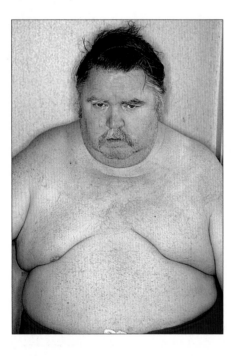

1 Grossly obese and cyanosed patient as he presented to the clinic.

QUESTIONS
1. What is the differential diagnosis and which is the most likely cause (*see* **2**)?
2. What investigation would establish the diagnosis?
3. What is the treatment?

Investigations

PaO_2:	6.1 kPa
$PaCO_2$:	8.8 kPa
pH:	7.23
Standard bicarbonate:	23.0 mmol/L
Urea:	16.7 mmol/L
Creatinine:	142 μmol/L
Electrolytes:	Normal

Respiratory function tests:

	Measured	Predicted
FEV_1:	1.75 L	56%
FVC:	2.05 L	50%
Residual volume (RV):	1.04 L	51.5%
Total lung capacity (TLC):	3.35 L	53.9%
$D_L co$:	21.2 ml/min/mmHg	78%

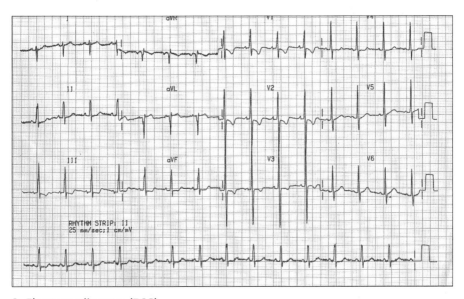

2 Electrocardiogram (ECG).

Case 2

ANSWERS

1. This gentleman's blood gases show type II respiratory failure with hypoxaemia and hypercapnia. His ECG (**2**) shows marked right ventricular hypertrophy. These features suggest that this man has developed cor pulmonale, which may be secondary to several possible primary diagnoses, such as:

   1) Obstructive sleep apnoea (OSA);
   2) Obesity hypoventilation (Pickwickian syndrome);
   3) Chronic obstructive pulmonary disease (COPD);
   4) Eisenmenger's syndrome.

   Eisenmenger's syndrome is unlikely in view of the raised $PaCO_2$. However, confirmation that an intracardiac shunt is not the cause of the hypoxaemia could be obtained by measuring the oxygen saturation when breathing 100% oxygen. In this gentleman's case, the oxygen saturation rose to 100% in response to this manoeuvre, excluding a shunt. If a significant shunt were present, it would not have been possible to increase the oxygen saturation above 90%. Chronic obstructive pulmonary disease(COPD) is not the cause of this gentleman's hypoxaemia, since his forced expiratory volume in one second (FEV_1) is well preserved (1.75 L). In general, COPD will not cause hypoxaemia if the FEV_1 is greater than 1 L.

   The likely diagnosis is a sleep-related breathing disorder, either OSA or obesity hypoventilation (OHV).

2. A recording of nocturnal oxygen saturation will confirm the diagnosis. Sleep studies vary in complexity from a recording of overnight oxygen saturation using a pulse oximeter to sophisticated polysomnographic recording systems, which also record chest and abdominal wall movement, naso-oral airflow, electro-encephalogram (EEG), electro-oculogram and submental electromyelogram (to define sleep stage). **3** shows the polysomnography results. There are repeated oxygen desaturations through the night which are most marked during rapid eye movement (REM) sleep (indicated in blue). The recording shows that most of the desaturations are due to obstructive apnoeas. Obstructive apnoeic episodes are more likely to occur during REM sleep since this is when skeletal muscle tone is lowest, predisposing to collapse of the pharynx and hypopharynx on inspiration. Patients with OSA usually complain of excessive daytime tiredness; this is the result of sleep fragmentation. Each obstructive apnoea is terminated by an arousal (awakening).The polysomnography summary opposite shows that the mean frequency of obstructive apnoeas was 85 per hour, and that the mean duration of each obstructive apnoea was 24.6 s. **4** shows a recording from an invasive sleep study, where respiratory effort was measured by an oesophageal balloon catheter system, airflow by a tight fitting face mask and sleep stage by an EEG. During an obstructive apnoea (when there is no airflow), there are increasing respiratory efforts until an increase in EEG amplitude occurs (an arousal) and the patient wakes momentarily. At this point, pharyngeal muscle tone is restored and airflow resumes, only to be followed by another apnoea.

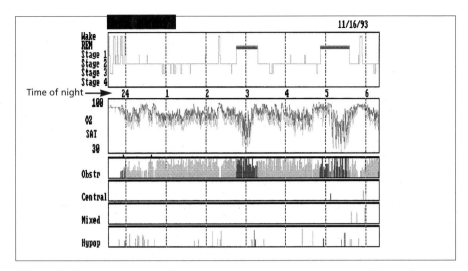

3 Results of polysomnography.

Polysomnography summary

	Obstructive	Mixed	Central	Hypopnoea
Total apnoeas:	556	3	3	31
Apnoeas per hour:	85	0.5	0.5	4.7
Mean apnoea: duration (s):	24.6	23.3	13.5	17.8

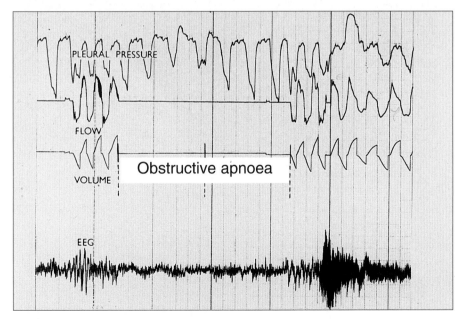

4 Invasive sleep study showing a series of six respiratory movements for which there is no airflow or volume change, despite pleural pressure swings.

13

Case 2

3. The usual management for OSA is nasal continuous positive airway pressure (CPAP) treatment at night when asleep (**5**). During sleep, upper airway muscle tone is reduced and the airway is prone to inspiratory collapse. Nasal CPAP provides the upper airway with a 'pneumatic splint', which prevents collapse during sleep. An alternative treatment is uvulopalatopharyngoplasty (UPPP). This operation involves removing part of the soft palate and uvula. Unfortunately, the site of upper airway collapse frequently involves the hypopharynx, which is not helped by upper airway surgery. Weight loss alone is rarely a successful treatment. Obstructive sleep apnoea can also occur in non-obese individuals. The illustration shows a patient wearing a CPAP mask. The pressure of the CPAP is adjusted until the upper airway obstructions are abolished; in the oximetry trace shown (**6**), the CPAP pressure was gradually increased until all apnoeas were abolished at a pressure of 14 cm H_2O.

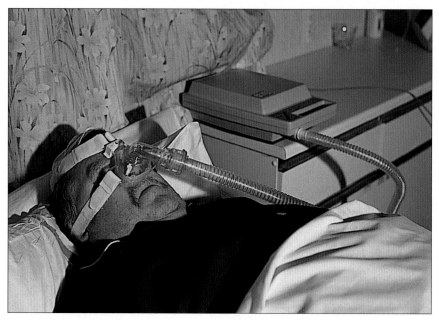

5 Patient on a CPAP machine.

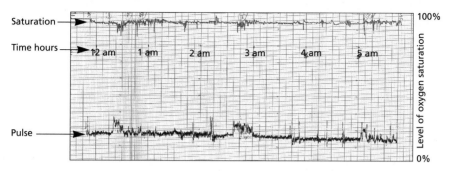

6 Post-CPAP treatment oximetry (saturation remains greater than 90% throughout the night).

Obesity hypoventilation, if not accompanied by a significant obstructive apnoea component, is best treated by nasal intermittent positive pressure ventilation (NIPPV), in which the ventilator cycles to augment both the depth and frequency of breathing during sleep.

Following one week's treatment with nasal CPAP set to 14 cm H$_2$O, the patient's nocturnal oxygen desaturations were abolished and his daytime hypoxaemia was improved. Also, he was no longer grossly hypercapnic. He had a much improved exercise tolerance, was able to manage a flight of stairs, and his breathlessness was reduced. His daytime hypersomnolence was no longer a problem. With continued treatment, his cor pulmonale should resolve.

Case 3
Chronic cough

A 59-year-old lady presented with a three-year history of a non-productive cough. The coughing bouts were more troublesome at night, but also occurred during the day. She did not complain of wheezing, dyspnoea or other chest symptoms. There was no past history of major illnesses; her only previous symptom was mild indigestion, and she had not smoked for 18 years (total exposure to cigarettes was one pack a day for 15 years). Treatment with many different types of cough linctus had been unsuccessful, and her symptoms continued to wake her and her husband at night.

On examination, the patient was obese, but no abnormal physical finding were elicited. The initial investigations were as follows:

Investigations

Haematology:	Haemoglobin (Hb): 11.4 g/dl
	White blood cell count (WBC):
	8.5 × 10⁹/L
	Eosinophils: 1.5 %
Spirometry:	FEV_1: 2.35 L (2.25)
	FVC: 2.95 L (3.38).
	(Predicted normals in brackets)
Skin prick tests:	Negative for common antigens
Radiology:	Chest radiograph (1)
	Sinus radiographs showed no abnormality

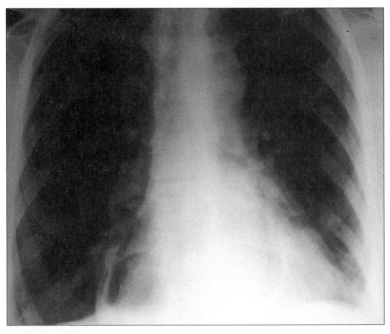

1 Chest radiograph.

Peak-flow monitoring showed normal values and no increase in diurnal variation. A bronchial challenge test was performed using a dosimeter. Doubling concentrations of histamine were delivered until the FEV_1 fell by 20% (PC_{20}). This occurred at a concentration of 16 mg/ml, which is a normal response and excludes increased bronchial hyper-reactivity. **2** shows the sound trace during a bout of coughing (plot of sound amplitude against time). The typical features of a 'peal' of five coughs are seen. Each cough shows two main peaks (*arrowed*) thought to be due to glottic opening and closing.

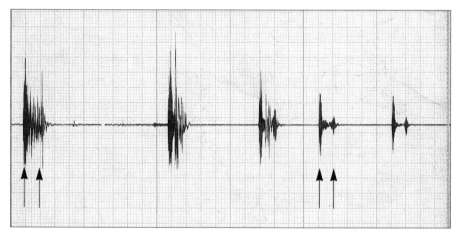

2 Sound trace during coughing.

QUESTIONS

1. What are the causes of chronic nocturnal cough in a patient without any obvious underlying chest disease?
2. What abnormality is shown in the chest radiograph (**1**)?
3. What other investigations would you arrange?
4. With the information given so far, what is the most likely diagnosis of this patient's complaint?
5. What treatment would you suggest?
6. List up to six non-pulmonary complications of chronic coughing.

Case 3

ANSWERS

1. Chronic nocturnal cough is most commonly associated with bronchial asthma or chronic obstructive airways disease. Some patients, particularly children, may have cough as the first presentation of allergic airways disease. Causes of cough at night in the absence of any known chest disease include chronic infection of the nose and sinuses (chronic post-nasal drip), incipient pulmonary oedema and gastro-oesophageal reflux.

2. The chest radiograph shows normal lung fields, but there is a shadow behind the heart. This retrocardiac, rounded 'mass' contains a fluid level, and has the characteristics of a hiatus hernia. A diagrammatic representation of the chest radiograph (1) is seen in 3.

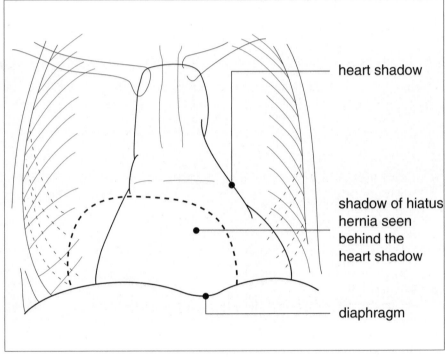

3 Diagrammatic representation of chest radiograph (**1**).

3. In view of the presence of a hiatus hernia, a barium meal was performed (**4**), which confirmed a sliding type of hiatus hernia associated with free oesophageal reflux. An oesophagoscopy and gastroscopy were also performed which, in addition to the hiatus hernia, demonstrated marked oesophagitis affecting the lower oesophagus (**5**). A more accurate method of assessing reflux, particularly if there is no hiatus hernia, is by the use of nocturnal oesophageal pH monitoring.

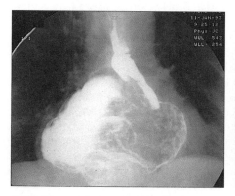
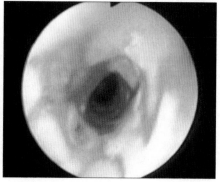

4 Radiograph showing barium meal.

5 Oesophagitis affecting lower oesophagus.

4. The most likely cause for this patient's nocturnal cough is the gastro-oesophageal reflux associated with a hiatus hernia. The reflux is always worse while lying flat at night, and this is thought to precipitate the bouts of coughing. In keeping with this presumptive diagnosis was the absence of any increase in bronchial hyperreactivity to histamine. However, this can at times be misleading, as asthma is occasionally precipitated by oesophageal reflux.

5. Treatment of the reflux was also used as a therapeutic trial. The administration of an H_2 antagonist (e.g. cimetidine or ranitidine), together with the recommended use of pillows in bed so as to sleep in a semi-recumbent posture, produced almost total relief of the patient's nocturnal cough. Occasionally, corrective surgery is required when the symptoms are very severe or do not respond to medical treatment.

6. There are various non-pulmonary complications of cough, including:
   - Cough fractures of the ribs;
   - Inguinal and femoral hernias;
   - Cough syncope (due to impaired venous filling of the heart);
   - Subconjunctival haemorrhage;
   - Uterine prolapse and stress incontinence;
   - Post-operative wound dehiscence.

Case 4
Asthma and a changing radiograph

A 39-year-old woman has had asthma since the age of 18. Her mother died of chronic asthma after many years of poor health. Initially her symptoms were mild, but these became very troublesome during her early 20s, with much coughing and sputum production. At the age of 27, she had her left upper lobe removed surgically after it had 'collapsed'. No further details are available. After the operation she enjoyed better health, got a job as a hotel receptionist and got married. She had no children, and kept no birds or furry pets. She had never smoked cigarettes, and drank little alcohol. In her early 30s she had an episode of right-sided pleurisy, but otherwise remained out of hospital while collecting regular bronchodilator and occasional inhaled steroid prescriptions from her doctor.

Two years before presentation she noticed a deterioration in her symptoms. She began to wake several nights each week with coughing and wheeze. She was breathless when carrying the shopping home, and was coughing 'dirty' sputum most days. In spite of taking inhaled steroid regularly and increasing the dose, she remained symptomatic. Then, over a period of a few weeks, she developed very green sputum with some blood staining, intermittent fevers with sweats, and her exercise tolerance decreased so that she was almost housebound. She was not cyanosed and was not distressed at rest. There was widespread expiratory wheezing, but no focal signs were noted in her chest to correspond with the changes on her radiograph (1). Blood tests showed an eosinophilia of 6% (of 7.2×10^9/L white cells) and an IgE level of >1000 IU/L. The FEV_1 was 2.2 L, and the FVC was 2.65 L (although she had taken her salbutamol just before), and the sputum culture was reported as 'mixed flora'. She was begun on a broad-spectrum antibiotic and asked to return in three weeks. At follow-up she was no better, and the chest radiograph was unchanged. She was referred to a respiratory unit, had further sputum and blood tests and a bronchoscopy, following which a diagnosis was made and treatment prescribed which dramatically improved both her symptoms and her chest radiograph. Over the next four years she was much better, but still had occasional exacerbations with temporary chest radiographic abnormalities. A radiograph from one of these episodes is shown (2), as are the original endobronchial biopsy (3—haematoxylin and eosin [H&E stain] and 4—Grocott's stain) and the dermal reaction to a specific antigen skin-prick test (5).

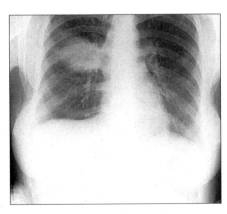

1 Initial PA chest radiograph.

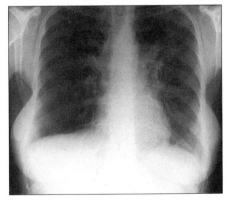

2 Chest radiograph showing shadowing on the contralateral side.

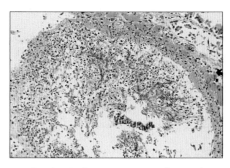

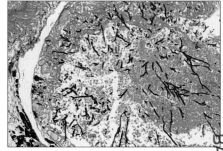

3 Histological appearance of samples obtained at bronchoscopy (H&E stain).

4 A similar specimen stained with Grocott's silver stain.

5 Dermal skin-prick test

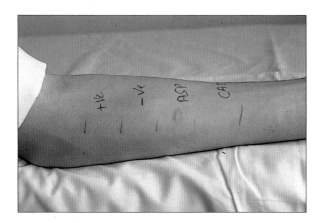

QUESTIONS

1. What is the diagnosis, and what does the biopsy show?
2. What did her physician write on the sputum request card?
3. What blood test did the physician request, and how does the information from the blood test differ from the antigen skin test of **4**?
4. How should the condition be treated, and what late complications may occur?

Case 4

ANSWERS

1. This lady has bronchopulmonary aspergillosis superimposed on bronchial asthma. The biopsy shows a mucous plug infiltrated with fungal hyphae of *Aspergillus fumigatus*. They are present on the H&E stain but much more apparent on the special silver stain, which clearly shows the typical branching filaments. Occasionally, it is possible to confirm positively the fungal species as *Aspergillus fumigatus* by finding the fruiting body of the organism (**6**). Colonisation of the airways by *Aspergillus* moulds is an unusual but well-recognised problem in asthma. The two main species of *Aspergillus*—*A. fumigatus* and *A. niger*—are both ubiquitous in the environment, and frequently colonise old buildings and air/ventilation ducts, especially areas in which there is damp and/or poor ventilation. The fungus may be found in the sputum of healthy people as a commensal, but in the immunocompromised patient, *Aspergillus* infection can become invasive within the lungs and can spread to other organs as invasive aspergillosis, which is difficult to treat effectively. In asthma, the *Aspergillus* usually remains localised within the bronchial tree and causes systemic upset via allergic mechanisms which manifest themselves as poorly controlled asthma and can include both early and late reactions. There are several different types of shadowing that can occur on the chest radiograph. An eosinophilic pneumonia may develop with appearances suggesting consolidation, as in the first radiograph of this lady. It is not infective and thus does not respond to antibiotics. At other times, mucous plugs develop, leading to either complete collapse of a lobe or appearing as thick opaque bronchi that resemble gloved fingers radiating from the hilum, as in **2**, or possibly resulting in thickened bronchial walls which appear as 'tramlines'. In each case, the allergic process usually responds well to oral corticosteroids. The diagnosis may only become apparent when a number of different patterns of lung shadowing in different sites is recognised.

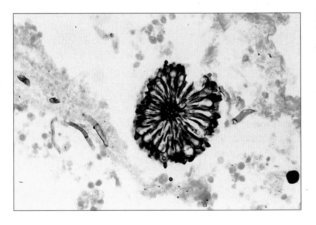

6 The head or 'fruiting body' of an *Aspergillus* mould.

2. Routine sputum samples are cultured for bacterial infection. Microbiological laboratory staff will not normally look for fungi in sputum unless specifically requested to do so on the request form. In this case, the physician asked the laboratory specifically to look for fungi in the sputum.

3. The blood test requested by the physician was for *Aspergillus* precipitins, i.e. the presence of specific IgG antibody to the *Aspergillus* antigen. The IgG class of antibody is associated with type 3 allergic reactions, which are typically associated with a late-phase (six to eight hours) asthma response. The presence of specific antibodies strongly suggests colonisation by the *Aspergillus* fungus but does not indicate whether this is bronchopulmonary infection or a chronic mycetoma. In contrast, the early (immediate) reaction is mediated by IgE, and can be detected with a dermal skin-prick test in which 0.1 ml of specific antigen and 0.1 ml of control saline are injected to different sites intradermally (4). A test is positive if the antigen (but not the control) results in a weal of greater than 3 mm in size within 15 minutes.

4. Anti-fungal agents do not penetrate sputum well, and the serum concentrations needed to treat *Aspergillus* in the airways are usually too toxic to be acceptable. In the immunocompromised, the risks of side-effects may be justifiable, but in asthma most patients can live acceptably with the fungus as long as the immunological responses are treated with steroids. High-dose oral prednisolone (30 mg/day) is needed to suppress the eosinophilic pulmonary infiltrates or to resolve the radiographic shadowing due to mucous plugging. Some patients need continuing low-dose oral steroids (5–7.5 mg/day) to maintain health, but in others steroids can be stopped (except for exacerbations) and the asthma controlled conventionally with inhaled steroids.

Late complications include progressive worsening of the airflow obstruction despite treatment; proximal cystic bronchiectasis; and the development of a fungal ball (mycetoma). The latter has the characteristic radiographic appearance of a discrete 'ball' sited within a lung cavity (7), but is sometimes only noted at postmortem (8).

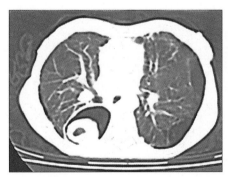

7 An aspergilloma radiographically.

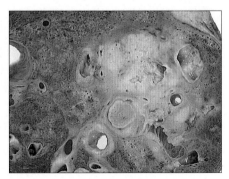

8 An aspergilloma pathologically.

Case 5
All that wheezes is not asthma

A 50-year-old man presented with recent onset of wheezing following an upper respiratory infection. For the past three years he had complained of a mild cough producing small amounts of clear sputum, but he had not previously noticed breathlessness during normal activities. Since the onset of his recent symptoms he had become dyspnoeic after walking approximately 100 yards or climbing one flight of stairs. There was no past history of any significant respiratory symptoms or other major illnesses or operations, but he had smoked 20 cigarettes daily since the age of 17. He did not keep any pets at home, had not suffered from hayfever and was unaware of any allergies. During his working life he had been employed in the ship-building industry, but he had never worked in the engine rooms. There was no family history of respiratory diseases.

On examination he looked well; there was no finger clubbing or palpable lymphadenopathy. He had a regular pulse rate of 84 beats per minute and a blood pressure of 160/90 mmHg. There was a mild wheeze audible at the mouth. Examination of his chest revealed normal expansion of the thoracic cage on inspiration, normal percussion and good air entry throughout both lung fields. On auscultation, expiratory wheezes were widely heard over the chest, together with an inspiratory wheeze on deep inspiration. The chest radiograph was normal.

The typical wheeze is seen in **1**. The sound trace is on the horizontal line; superimposed on this is a flow trace, the upward deflection representing expiration and the downward, inspiration. When this sound is analysed by frequency using sophisticated digital signal processing techniques, a three-dimensional image of the sound can be made (**2**). **2** shows a wheeze which falls in frequency during inspiration as airway geometry alters.

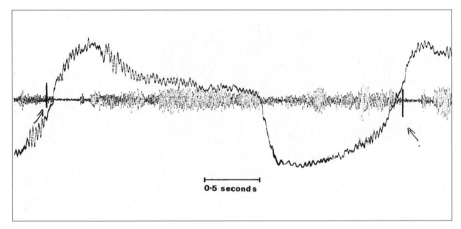

0·5 seconds

1 Sound trace (horizontal line) and flow trace (superimposed line) of a typical wheeze. The upward deflection represents expiration and the downward deflection represents inspiration.

Case 5

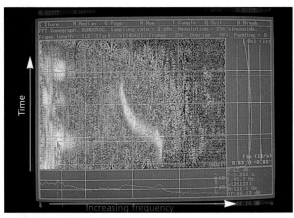

2 Three-dimensional colour image created by analysis of wheeze sound frequency using digital signal processing techniques. Time is represented on the vertical and frequency on the horizontal axis; power is represented by colour (yellow = highest intensity; blue = lowest intensity).

Investigations:

FEV_1:	1.5 L (predicted 2.6 L)
FVC:	2.6 L (predicted 3.75 L)
FEV_1 %:	57%
Flow–volume loop:	(*see* 3)
Hb:	15.7 g/dl
WBC:	10.8×10^9/L
	(72% neutrophils, 23% lymphocytes, 1% eosinophils)
IgE:	5 IU/L

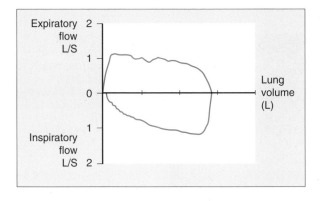

3 Flow-volume loop.

QUESTIONS
1. What does the simple spirometry show (FEV_1, FVC and FEV_1 %)?
2. What diagnoses are usually associated with this type of spirometric abnormality?
3. From the history and initial investigations, what is the most likely diagnosis, and what other pulmonary function test should be performed?
4. What does the flow-volume loop show (**3**), and does this suggest an alternative diagnosis?
5. What other investigations should be considered to confirm this suspicion?
6. What treatments are available for this condition?

Case 5

ANSWERS

1. The spirometry shows evidence of airflow obstruction (a low FEV_1 with a relatively well-preserved FVC). Normally the FEV_1 is at least 70% of the FVC, but, as in this case, in airflow obstruction the FEV_1 percentage is reduced.

2. The main causes of airflow obstruction are bronchial asthma, chronic bronchitis/emphysema (chronic obstructive pulmonary disease [COPD]) and a localised main airway obstruction.

3. The history of a recent onset of wheezing in a patient with no significant past respiratory symptoms could suggest late-onset asthma, but in a smoker, COPD cannot be ruled out since patients often overlook early mild symptoms for many years. The way to diagnose asthma is to demonstrate variability of over 15% in the FEV_1 or peak flow, either spontaneously or after inhaled bronchodilators. In this patient, 5 mg of nebulised salbutamol did not produce any improvement in the FEV_1 and the peak-flow charts showed no variation. Before assuming a diagnosis of COPD, however, the flow-volume loop should be examined.

4. The flow-volume loop shows attenuation and alteration in the shape of both the expiratory and inspiratory loops which is characteristic of a fixed intrathoracic obstruction. In asthma and COPD, the sharp expiratory peak is preserved and the inspiratory loop may be somewhat attenuated, but it maintains its typical semi-circular shape. Thus, the flow-volume loop suggests the probability of an obstructing lesion such as a tumour in the trachea or the main carina.

5. The investigation of choice is a bronchoscopy. In this case, a fibre-optic bronchoscopy was performed under local anaesthesia and showed a polypoid and infiltrating tumour at the main carina, reducing the diameter of the airway to approximately one-third of its normal size. 4 is a photograph of these changes. A biopsy was taken, and the tumour was subsequently reported as a squamous-cell carcinoma.

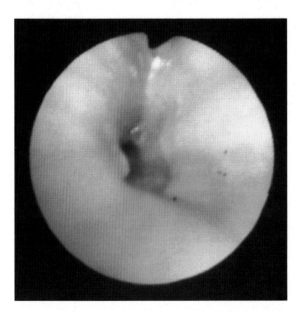

4 A polypoid and infiltrating tumour at the main carina, which has reduced the diameter of the airway to one-third of its normal size.

6. This tumour is inoperable, as surgery is not possible with a carcinoma involving the main carina. In addition, such tumours usually involve the surrounding mediastinal tissues. The usual treatment option is external beam radiotherapy, but caution is required with critical stenosis as oedema after radiotherapy can cause major life-threatening airway obstruction. In these circumstances, the tumour can be debulked endoscopically, using either diathermy or laser treatments. An alternative approach is the use of expandable metal stents which can be introduced endoscopically either before radiotherapy or when the disease progresses. In this case, radiotherapy alone was used with initial alleviation of symptoms. However, within three months the airway became critically narrowed, with almost complete occlusion of the left main bronchus, resulting in a very distressing recurrence of severe dyspnoea. At this time, stents were introduced endobronchially into the right main bronchus, resulting in the rapid relief of symptoms. **5** and **6** show the radiographic appearances before and after the placement of the stents. The metal coils are easily seen. The patient died a month later without the distressing symptom of asphyxiation. A further treatment option currently being evaluated in specialist centres is endobronchial radiotherapy (brachy therapy), which can be coupled with the use of stenting.

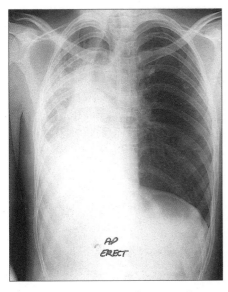

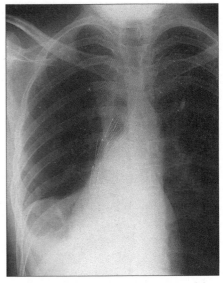

5 Chest radiograph before stenting introduced.

6 Chest radiograph after stents introduced into left main bronchus. Note metal coils in place.

Case 6
Breathlessness and big toes

A 50-year-old sewage maintenance worker attended hospital for left-sided chest pain following a blow to the chest at work. His ninth rib was fractured, but the radiologist noted additional pulmonary shadowing and suggested referral to hospital outpatients. Some months later he attended, and a history of increasing breathlessness over the past few years was obtained. He had smoked 50 cigarettes per day until his work accident, but had never been troubled by wheezing or sputum production. However, he had had a dry irritating cough for some months. He could walk about 100 yards on level ground but found he could only climb stairs if he took his time. His present job included digging manholes, and this was proving difficult for him. His father had died of lung cancer and his brother had recently had a coronary artery bypass graft, so he was concerned that he too might have heart disease. He had no other symptoms, and in particular no history of joint disease. On examination he was markedly breathless on simply undressing, but was not cyanosed. His toes are shown in **1**. He had no heart murmurs, and the jugular venous pulse was not elevated. In the chest there was no audible wheeze, but there were showers of mid-to-late fine inspiratory crackles. His chest radiograph (**2**) was abnormal, and so too were the CT scan (**3**) and lung function tests (*see* **Investigations** and **4**). Arterial blood gases showed a PaO_2 of 8.2 kPa and a $PaCO_2$ of 4.5 kPa. An ECG was normal.

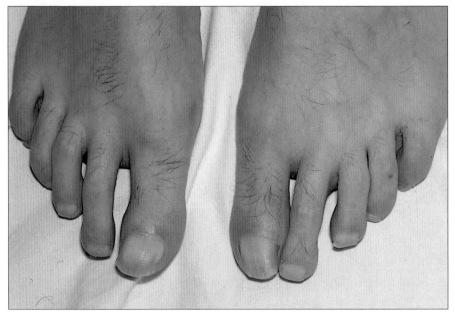

1 Photograph of patient's feet.

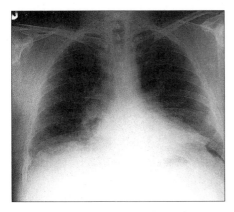

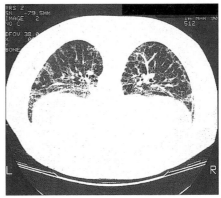

2 Plain chest radiograph from four years earlier.

3 CT scan.

Investigations

	Actual	Predicted
FEV$_1$:	2.4 L	2.9 L
FEV$_1$ post-salbutamol :	2.5 L	
Forced vital capacity:	2.8 L	3.8 L
Residual volume (helium dilution):	1.5 L	1.8 L
Total lung capacity (helium):	4.3 L	5.7 L
D$_L$co	12.3 ml/min/mmHg	25 ml/min/mmHg

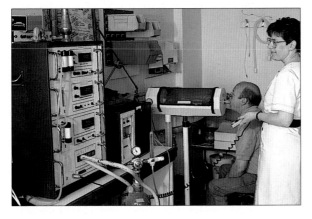

4 D$_L$co measurement.

QUESTIONS
1. What is the differential diagnosis?
2. How would you confirm the diagnosis?
3. What is the prognosis?
4. What treatments might you consider, and how would you monitor the outcome?

Case 6

1. The diagnosis in this man is fibrosing alveolitis. The evidence for this is clinical (finger clubbing and basal inspiratory lung crackles on auscultation), radiographic (basal shadowing on the chest radiograph and sub-pleural crescents on the high-resolution CT scan) and physiological (total lung capacity less than 80% predicted and diffusing capacity ($D_L$co) less than 50% predicted). There is no cardiac enlargement or upper lobe blood diversion on the radiograph to suggest heart failure. The differential diagnosis concerns the aetiology of the lung fibrosis. There are no symptoms or signs to suggest a connective tissue disease or sarcoidosis, and he had never worked with asbestos or other fibrogenic dusts. Thus, in the absence of an identifiable cause, it is probable that this is cryptogenic fibrosing alveolitis (CFA).

2. The only way to be quite sure of the diagnosis is to perform a lung biopsy. Fibre-optic transbronchial biopsies are difficult to interpret because they are so small, and most chest physicians would request an open-lung biopsy under direct vision. This always used to require a limited thoracotomy with its associated morbidity, but modern technology means that a keyhole approach is possible (using video-assisted thoracoscopy). This provides a substantial sample for the pathologist, with minimal morbidity for the patient. This man's histology (**5**) shows extensive fibrosis of his alveoli with no asbestos bodies. There is little inflammation and, significantly, no evidence of arteritis or granuloma formation.

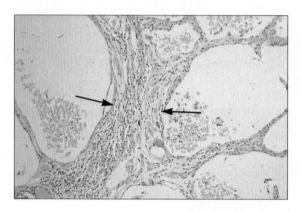

5 Histology. There is marked thickening of the alveolar interstitium (*arrowed*) with inflammatory cell infiltrate and collagen deposition.

3. The prognosis of CFA is very variable. In its most acute form (Hamman–Rich syndrome), the symptoms develop over a few weeks and can progress to respiratory failure and death within six months. More typically, progress is less aggressive, and overall the median survival has been reported to be 54 months. Factors associated with a worse outcome include male sex, a high profusion of radiographic shadowing, high intensity of breathlessness and a low cellularity on the lung biopsy. This man would seem to be in the worse category on each count. **6** shows a post-mortem specimen of a whole lung with marked bossellation of the pleural surface. The section of the lung is seen in **7**, which shows extensive fibrosis with honeycombe changes.

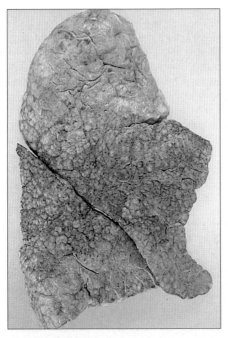 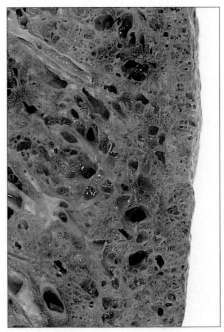

6 Bosselated lung surface.

7 Cut section of bosselated lung.

4. There is no uniformly successful treatment for CFA. High-dose oral corticosteroids are usually tried in the hope that they will suppress the inflammatory
process within the lung (7) and thus arrest progress. Patients with a high degree
of cellularity on their biopsies are said to respond best. If there is a response, then
oral steroids can be continued either alone or with other immuno-modulatory
agents. The best documented of these is cyclophosphamide in low doses (50 or
100 mg/day). If these agents do not work, then the only other approach is to
consider lung transplantation. In a patient at 50 years of age with progressive
deterioration and thus a poor prognosis, this is justifiable. However, only a few
such patients will ever receive a transplant because the supply of donor lungs
and the ability to transplant them remain limited. Thus it is inadvisable for
patients to have their hopes unduly raised.

Monitoring the effect of treatment is best done by objective serial recording
of lung function. The forced vital capacity (FVC) and the diffusing capacity for
carbon monoxide ($D_L$co) are the most useful. Symptoms are less reliable,
particularly in assessing the results of oral steroid therapy, because of the
temporary euphoriant effect of steroids. At 36 months, this man was still alive but
was deteriorating. His lung function tests had been entirely unchanged after
steroids and eight months of low-dose cyclophosphamide, and thereafter his lung
function had slowly declined to an FVC of 2.2 L (56% predicted) and a $D_L$co of
36% (predicted). He was much more breathless and hypoxic at rest (PaO_2 6.3
kPa). Conservative treatment was continuing with the addition of an oxygen
concentrator at home.

Case 7
The smoker's curse

A 58-year-old man who had a chronic productive cough due to smoking 20 cigarettes daily since he was 18 years old developed a sore throat, and his sputum became purulent. He noticed that he had become a little breathless on climbing the stairs, and, on several occasions after bouts of coughing, his sputum contained a few streaks of blood. He sought medical advice and was diagnosed as having an acute exacerbation of chronic bronchitis, for which he was given a course of amoxycillin. His sputum rapidly cleared, but about one month later he complained of some back pain and noticed further streaking of blood in his sputum. A chest radiograph with a lateral view was arranged, and results are seen in **1** and **2**. On examination he looked well and had no finger clubbing or palpable lymphadenopathy, but a few inspiratory crackles were heard over the left upper lobe on examination of his chest.

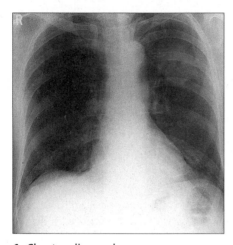

1 Chest radiograph.

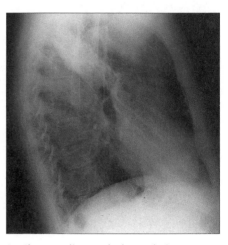

2 Chest radiograph, lateral view.

In the past he had suffered from a myocardial infarction, and had subsequently complained of mild-effort angina which was well controlled with medication, but he had had no other illnesses. He was employed as a taxi driver. This patient was sent to his local hospital chest clinic, where the following investigations were arranged:

Investigations

Hb:	12.8 g/dl
ESR:	66 mm in one hour
Urea:	4.5 mmol/L
Electrolytes were within normal limits	
Resting ECG (**3**) showed inverted T-waves in leads II, III, aVF and V4–6	
FEV_1 was 1.8 L and FVC was 2.8 L, giving an $FEV_1\%$ of 64	

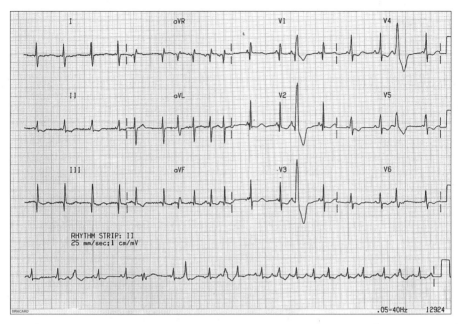

3 ECG.

QUESTIONS

1. What was the presumptive diagnosis in this case? What do the chest radiographs (**1** and **2**) show?
2. What definitive investigation would you perform, and what precautions would you take before initiating this investigation?
3. What is the preferred treatment, and what criteria have to be met before such treatment can be offered?
4. What are the alternative treatments?
5. What is the overall prognosis for this condition?

Case 7

ANSWERS

1. The presumptive diagnosis in any smoker who develops haemoptysis is carcinoma of the bronchus. This assumption was made more likely by the chest radiograph, which showed an ill-defined mass in the left upper zone. The lateral view confirmed this to be in the upper lobe. The chest radiograph also shows some fractured healed ribs on the right side. Pathological fractures were excluded by a bone scan which, in this case, was reported as normal.

2. The definitive investigation is a bronchoscopy. Bronchoscopy can be performed under a general anaesthetic with the rigid instrument or under a local anaesthetic with a fibrescope. Before undertaking a bronchoscopy, it is usual to perform a vitalograph, and if the FEV_1 is reduced to 1 L or below, blood gases should be estimated. Haemoglobin, urea and electrolyte and a prothombin time should be measured. Caution is needed if the ECG is ischaemic; bronchoscopy is not advised for at least eight weeks after a myocardial infarction. In this case, there were no contra-indications to bronchoscopy (**4**), and a tumour was demonstrated arising from the left upper lobe. A biopsy was taken (**5**), which showed changes characteristic of a squamous-cell carcinoma.

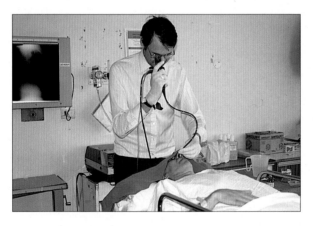

4 Fibre-optic examination being performed.

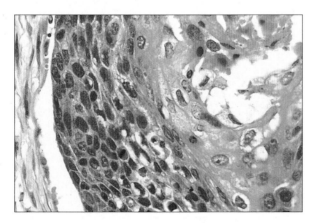

5 Biopsy showing squamous-cell carcinoma.

3. The preferred treatment is surgical resection; however, in order for a tumour to be resectable, the following main criteria have to be met:

a) The trachea, main carina and upper part of the main bronchus on the affected side must be clear of tumour.
b) There should be no evidence of significant lymphadenopathy or invasion of tumour into the mediastinum on a CT scan. Any equivocal glands, if accessible, should be examined by mediastinoscopy.
c) There should be no evidence of secondary spread to the liver or adrenal glands on CT scanning of the abdomen.
d) There should be no evidence of other secondary spread, and if there is any bone pain, a bone scan should be performed.
e) The cardiopulmonary systems should have sufficient reserve to withstand resection and the trauma of the peri-operative period.

In this case the tumour was resectable at bronchoscopy. The CT seen in **6** did not show any mediastinal lymphadenopathy, and the bone scan was normal. Although the patient had suffered a previous myocardial infarction and had mild airflow obstruction, he had enough cardiopulmonary reserve to undergo surgery. He successfully underwent a left upper lobectomy. The resected tumour is seen in **7**.

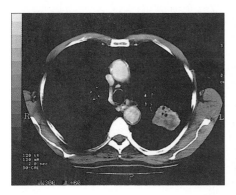
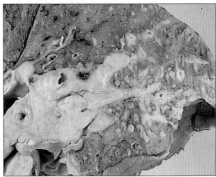

6 CT scan.   **7** Resected tumour.

4. The only curative treatment for squamous-cell carcinoma is surgery. Radical radiotherapy is the only alternative to surgery; but controlled trials have confirmed that surgical results are better. It is only suitable for patients who are medically unfit for surgery. For non–small-cell tumours that are not resectable, amelioration of distressing symptoms can be achieved with palliative radiotherapy. These symptoms include main airway obstruction, haemoptysis, superior veno-caval obstruction, and chest wall or bone pain, amelioration of distressing symptoms can be achieved with radiotherapy. However, secondary deposits in the liver or brain are not greatly helped by radiotherapy.
5. The overall survival rate for non–small-cell lung cancer is very poor, being only 4–7% at five years. Unfortunately, this figure has not altered in the last 30 years. Following surgery, the average five-year survival rate is 25%, and at 10 years, 16–18%.

Case 8
"Lily the Pink"

A 32-year-old woman with previously good health complained of general tiredness and lassitude and had lost a few kg in weight. She developed a mild, non-productive cough and occasionally complained of an aching on the right side of her chest. Since the age of 15 she had smoked between 15 and 20 cigarettes per day.

On examination she looked fit; there was no finger clubbing or significant lymphadenopathy. Examination of her chest revealed no abnormal signs, and abdominal and neurological examinations were similarly normal. A chest radiograph was performed by her general practitioner, and the results found to be abnormal (**1**). She was therefore referred to her local hospital outpatient department, where the following investigations were performed:

Investigations

Hb:	11.2 g/dl
WBC:	8.5×10^9/L
Differential count:	Normal
Urea:	4.6 mmol/L
Electrolytes:	Normal
Repeat chest radiograph:	Unchanged from **1**
	Lateral view seen in **2**
Abdominal ultrasound:	Normal
FEV$_1$:	2.5 L (predicted 3.0 l)
FVC:	3.1 L (predicted 3.8 l)
FEV$_1$ %:	80%

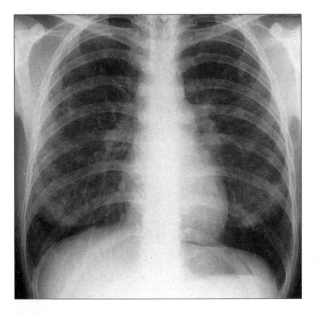

1 Chest radiograph showing abnormalities.

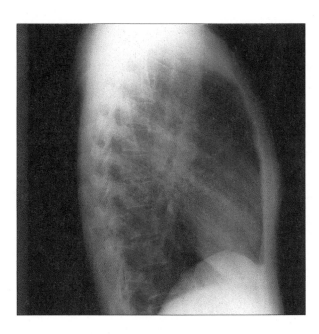

2 Chest radiograph, lateral view.

As the diagnosis was not established on the basis of the initial history, examination or investigations, a bronchoscopy and transbronchial biopsy were performed. The bronchoscopy was normal, and the small amount of biopsy material revealed only some non-specific inflammatory changes. Subsequently, an open-lung biopsy was performed through a limited thoracotomy. A representative section of the lung tissue is seen in the photomicrograph (**3**). This shows many irregularly shaped histiocytic cells, together with an infiltration of other cells, particularly eosinophils.

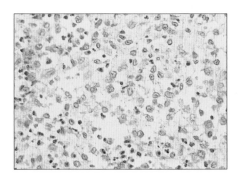

3 Section of lung tissue.

QUESTIONS

1. Describe the abnormalities on the chest radiograph.
2. What is the most likely cause for the radiographic appearances? Describe how pulmonary nodular disease is classified.
3. What was the diagnosis in this case?
4. What non-pulmonary features may be present?
5. What is the prognosis, and what complications may occur?
6. Would you start any treatment?

Case 8

1. The chest radiograph shows reticulo-nodular shadowing throughout both lung fields. The nodular opacities are between 3 and 10 mm in diameter, and there is relative sparing of both costophrenic angles. There is no evidence on the plain films of mediastinal lymphadenopathy, although CT scanning would be required to confirm this. Multiple nodular opacities on the chest radiograph have many causes; some of the most common of these are seen in **Table 1.**

Table 1   Multiple pulmonary nodules

- Bronchial carcinoma
- Metastatic carcinoma (most commonly adenocarcinoma)
- Lymphomas
- Granulomatous disease (tuberculosis, sarcoidosis, Wegener's, eosinophilic)
- Pneumoconiosis
- Rheumatoid disease (nodules)
- Acute infections (multiple abscesses)
- Fungal infections (coccidioidomycosis, histoplasmosis)

2. The most likely cause for nodular opacities of this size on a chest radiograph is a metastatic tumour. The usual histology in a young woman would be secondary adenocarcinoma of breast, gastrointestinal or ovarian origin. However, metastatic disease is uncommon in a 32-year-old, and rarer causes of such shadowing have to be considered. The diagnosis is almost always made by histological examination of lung tissue. Transbronchial biopsy only provides small-tissue specimens, and, while these are sufficient to diagnose carcinoma or sarcoidosis, it is unusual for them to provide adequate tissue for the rarer diagnoses. In these difficult cases, an open biopsy or, more recently, a thorascopic biopsy, must be performed.

3. The histology in this case does not show any malignant cells. There is a mixture of histiocytes, eosinophils and granulomata (3), which is characteristic of pulmonary eosinophilic granulomatosis. Electron microscopy showed diagnostic Birbeck granules. This is a condition of unknown aetiology, and is grouped under the overall heading of histiocytosis X. Other associated diseases are Hand–Schüller–Christian disease and Letterer–Siwe disease, both of which occur in a younger age group and are more often associated with extra-pulmonary manifestations.

4. Non-pulmonary features of this condition are fever, weight loss and malaise (as in this case). Lytic lesions in bone are seen (the examples in **4** and **5** are not from this patient). Any other system may be involved, but this is more common in other varieties of histiocytosis X.

5. The prognosis is very variable, and to a large extent depends on the pulmonary complications. If the disease is progressive, there is gradual deterioration of pulmonary function over 5–15 years. The radiograph gradually changes to produce multiple small-ring shadows, resulting in 'honeycomb' lung; later, larger cysts and bullae develop. At this stage pneumothorax is common and difficult to treat. Eventually, death results from respiratory failure. Bad prognostic features are multisystem disease, honeycombing on the radiograph, recurrent pneumo-thoraces, reduced diffusing capacity ($D_L co$) on pulmonary function testing and the onset of the disease in old age. If none of these complications is present,

prognosis is good. Some patients experience a remission, including this patient, whose current radiograph is seen in **6** (note that the clips used for the lung biopsy are clearly seen at the left base).

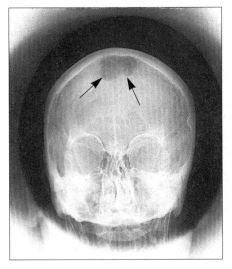

4 Lytic lesions seen on cranial bone.

5 Lytic lesions seen on cranial bone.

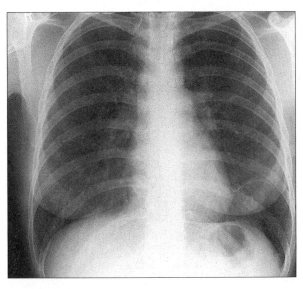

6 Patient's current chest radiograph, with the clips used for the lung biopsy visible at left base.

6. Many treatments have been tried, including steroids and immunosuppressive drugs. The evidence for their efficacy is anecdotal, based on single cases. Treatment of complications should be undertaken. Pneumothorax can be treated with pleurodesis or pleurectomy, but caution is needed in treating young patients for whom a lung transplant might become a possibility, as such procedures would make subsequent transplantation difficult. Respiratory failure is treated in the standard way, and patients may require domiciliary oxygen.

Case 9
Acute severe dyspnoea

A 39-year-old man (1) presents to the casualty department at 11.00 pm. He is severely breathless, and describes his story in broken sentences. He developed an upper respiratory infection four days previously and has become progressively unwell since. The previous night he had hardly slept because he was coughing so much. However, he produced only small amounts of thick white sputum. He has never had anything like this before. The doctor noted his distressed breathing and that there were few signs on auscultation, and the patient's colour was good although an oxygen mask was in place. A peak-flow meter was handed to the patient, who was unable to register a reading at all. His wife reported that he was a non-smoker who had been a very fit, sport-loving person in the past, but she had noticed that he had not been very active for the last two years or so and had been coughing and pausing during simple domestic tasks such as mowing the lawn. She had noticed that he had been wheezing while asleep for the past week or so and occasionally before that.

Nebulised drugs were begun (2) and an arterial blood sample taken (3), and the doctor prescribed one of the two drugs in 4. Twenty minutes later he was visibly more relaxed, talked comfortably and asked to go home.

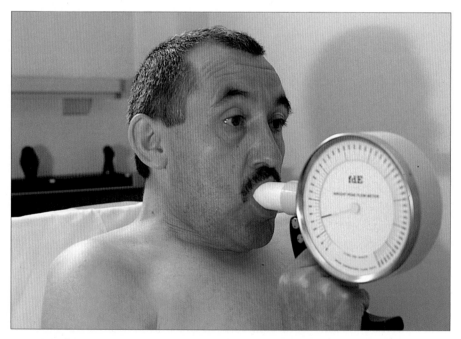

1 Patient being assessed on arrival in casualty. The oxygen mask has been removed for a moment to let him blow into a peak expiratory flow (PEF) meter.

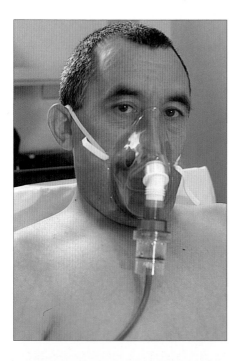

2 Patient with oxygen mask in place looking more relaxed after a nebuliser.

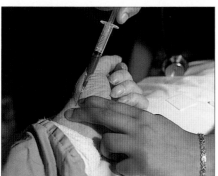

3 Arterial blood gases being taken from the radial artery.

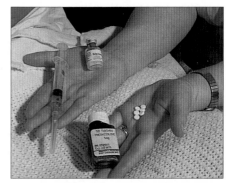

4 Prednisolone tablets or intravenous hydrocortisone?

QUESTIONS

1. What features might suggest asthma rather than another cause of respiratory distress?
2. Why should you admit him in spite of the response to treatment?
3. What are the results of the blood gas analysis likely to show? What values would cause you to be concerned, and why?
4. What treatment would you give now and in what order?
5. How would you assess the efficacy of the immediate treatments, and at what time?
6. What advice would you give this man for the future, once his acute attack was over?

Case 9

ANSWERS

1. The relatively short history is typical of asthma, but it could be an acute infection. Cough is a common feature of asthma. Although patients may not describe wheeze spontaneously, on specific questioning their spouses may have noticed wheezing, especially at night. The symptoms of acute distress, being unable to complete sentences, absent or very faint breath sounds and being unable to register anything on a peak-flow meter strongly suggest asthma, and should be treated as such in the first instance. Acute infections with this degree of respiratory distress are likely to be associated with a pyrexia and with an abnormal chest radiograph, but acute therapy should not be withheld pending the radiograph.

2. Patients may often respond dramatically to nebulised bronchodilators and ask to be sent home straight away. In this case, the degree of distress was marked, there were signs of potentially life-threatening asthma (silent chest and inability to speak in sentences) and the peak flow was very, very low. Each alone would justify admission, since the effect of the nebuliser is likely to wear off after three to four hours, leaving the patient back to square one or worse. In addition, this man can be expected to deteriorate during the night, as the diurnal peak-flow values reach their physiological nadir at around 4.00 am.

3. The arterial blood gases showed the following:

pH:	7.32
PaO_2:	17.4 kPa
$PaCO_2$:	5.5 kPa
Bicarbonate:	25 mmol/L.

   These were taken when the patient was already on oxygen—hence the raised PaO_2. Since most ambulance services will have begun oxygen as they collect the patient, it is now unusual to detect hypoxia in acute asthma. This should not lull the physician into a false sense of security—particularly when, as in this case, it would appear that the pH and $PaCO_2$ are both normal. McFadden showed 20 years ago that 75% of asthma patients present with a low carbon dioxide tension, and that a normal level or a raised level is an indication that the patient is becoming tired and is very likely to require intermittent positive pressure ventilation (IPPV) unless he responds well to initial therapy.

4. Initial treatment consists of oxygen (in the highest concentration available), nebulised bronchodilators (e.g.salbutamol, 5 mg and ipratropium bromide, 500 μg in combination in the same nebuliser) and high-dose systemic steroids. There has been much debate as to whether intravenous steroids work faster than oral tablets, but the consensus now suggests there is no real difference—either can be prescribed. Although intravenous drugs reach the circulation faster, it takes up to six hours by either route for medication to penetrate the cells and begin to modify the inflammatory reaction.

5. The response to the initial bronchodilators must be monitored by repeating the peak-flow readings 15–30 minutes after the dose. The results should be plotted on a chart, and if the patient is improving, bronchodilators can be repeated at four-to-six hourly intervals together with further peak expiratory flow readings. This provides an objective record of progress (5). If the patient is not improving, the nebuliser can be repeated sooner, or intravenous aminophylline considered. In this case the normal $PaCO_2$ is a potential cause for alarm, and the blood gases too should be repeated or oxygen saturation monitored continuously with an oximeter. A rising $PaCO_2$ or a falling pH despite therapy points towards the need for immediate IPPV.

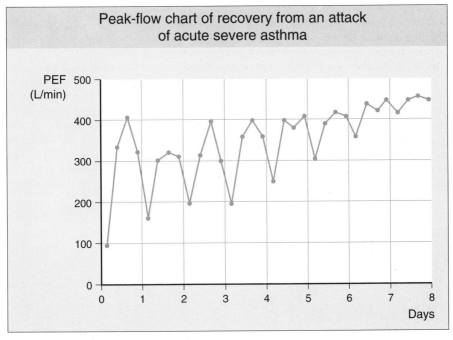

Peak-flow chart of recovery from an attack of acute severe asthma

5 Peak-flow chart during recovery.

6. Planning this man's future care is probably the most important part of the whole admission. Two-thirds of asthma admissions are readmissions, and as such might have been potentially preventable. Advice should include how to use inhalers, when to take the different types of inhalers and how to monitor, record and interpret the PEF readings (**6**). Asthma audit shows that this planning of future management is not done well by many hospitals, yet this is the opportunity to teach the patient about asthma, and how he can both control ongoing symptoms and prevent further admissions.

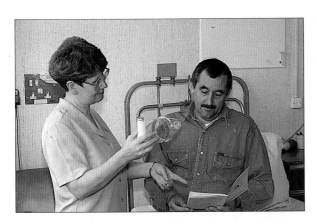

6 Patient having his inhaler technique checked on the ward and an individualised self-management plan set out by an asthma specialist nurse.

Case 10
A multi-system problem

A 52-year-old woman was referred by her general practitioner to the chest clinic because of breathlessness after walking approximately 300 yards on level ground. She had a chronic, irritating, non-productive cough but no other chest symptoms. She had been a life-long non-smoker. Other complaints included parasthesia of both hands, mild arthritis of the interphalangeal joints and some recent weight loss.

On examination she was not breathless at rest, and there was no audible wheezing. She was thin and had a 'rash' around her mouth (**1**). Her hands were abnormal, as seen in **2**, but there was no swelling of any joints. Neurological examination revealed impairment of light touch, pinprick-like sensations extending to both wrists and some wasting of the small muscles of both hands. On examination of her chest there was reduced percussion at both bases, and on auscultation there were some abnormal signs which were best heard at the lung bases and in the axillae.

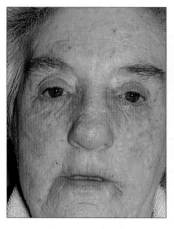

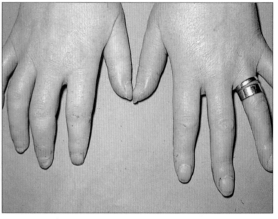

1 'Rash' around patient's mouth and on her face.

2 Patient's hands showing signs of abnormality. On examination these were found to have wasting of the small muscles.

Investigations

Hb:	13.6 g/dl
WBC:	10.5×10^9/L
ESR:	50 mm in first hour
Urea:	6.3 mmol/L
Pulmonary function tests, with predicted normals in brackets, were as follows:	
FEV_1:	1.4 L (2.8)
FVC:	1.8 L (2.3)
FEV_1 %:	77%

A CT scan of her chest was subsequently performed, and a representative high-resolution section from the lung base is seen in **3**. Her chest radiograph is seen in **4**.

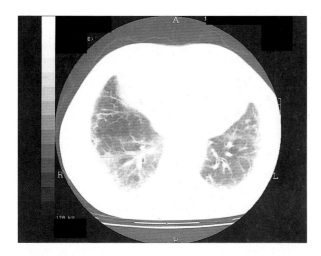

3 CT scan.

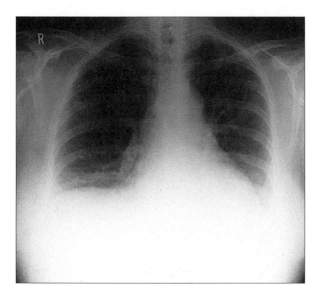

4 Chest radiograph.

QUESTIONS
1. Describe the abnormality on the hands and face and give the likely diagnosis. Suggest two other symptoms that this patient is likely to have.
2. List the abnormalities on the chest radiograph and CT scan.
3. What is the classical physical sign heard in the chest with this abnormality, and why does this occur?
4. What are the abnormalities on the pulmonary function tests?
5. What other investigations should be considered?
6. What treatments are available?

Case 10

ANSWERS

1. The mouth is small and puckered with perioral telangiectasia. The hands show tight, indurated skin resulting in a flexure deformity, and the fingertips are deformed. The changes around the mouth and sclerodactyly are classical symptoms of systemic sclerosis. Additional symptoms in this patient included severe Raynaud's phenomenon and persistent symptoms of reflux oesophagitis.

2. The chest radiograph shows irregular reticulo-nodular shadowing maximal in the lower zones. The high-resolution CT scan shows the shadowing in more detail. The peripheral areas of the lung are more affected than the central area, the maximal shadowing being just below the surface of the lung. These changes in the lungs are typical of diffuse interstitial pulmonary fibrosis, in this case secondary to systemic sclerosis.

   An open-lung biopsy confirmed the diagnosis of fibrosing alveolitis (**5**). There are no pathognomonic pathological features to indicate its association with scleroderma.

3. The classical physical sign in the chest is inspiratory lung crackles. A typical phonopneumographic tracing of crackles is seen (**6**). On the tracing, the horizontal line is the sound trace, showing several 'spikes' which are individual crackles. They occur at the end of inspiration as indicated by the flow trace. Crackles occur particularly in conditions in which the lungs are stiff. In these circumstances, the smaller airways collapse on expiration; on breathing in, a differential pressure develops across these collapsed airways, and when of sufficient magnitude (usually towards the end of inspiration), the airway snaps open. The sudden equalisation of downstream and upstream pressure is thought to be the most likely cause for the crackling sound. The crackles are fine- and late-inspiratory, and are often perceived as high-pitched. As the disease progresses, the crackles become more profuse and fill more of the inspiration.

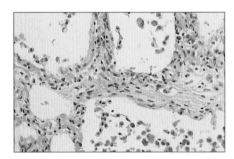

5 Open-lung biopsy.

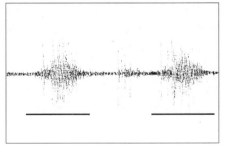

6 Typical phonopneumographic tracing of crackles. The spikes on the horizontal line are individual crackles in the second half of inspiration (marked by solid bar).

4. The pulmonary function tests show a restrictive defect of ventilation (reduced FEV_1 and FVC giving a normal FEV_1/FVC ratio of 70%). The transfer or diffusing capacity ($D_L co$) is reduced in keeping with an interstitial process.

5. The diagnosis is usually apparent on physical examination. Immunological markers are common, circulating antinuclear antibodies (usually of the speckled or nucleolar pattern) being found in virtually all patients. A search for other organ involvement is important as the prognosis is much worse if there is evidence of cardiac, renal or pulmonary involvement. Involvement of the gut, particularly the oesophagus, is common, and a barium meal is usually administered. **7** and **8** show an atonic oesophagus with free reflux.

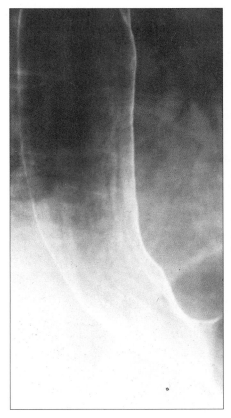

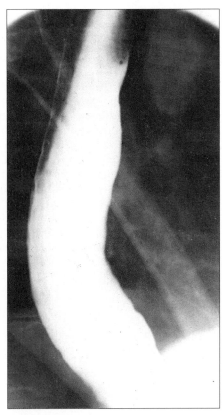

7 Radiograph showing atonic oesophagus.

8 Radiograph showing atonic oesophagus with free reflux.

6. Treatment of systemic sclerosis is unsatisfactory. General care of the skin is important, and vasodilators are often used to improve the microcirculation. Overall, anti-inflammatory drugs do not seem very useful; however, fibrosing alveolitis is usually treated with steroids. Steroids were prescribed in this case, and the disease has not progressed, but it is difficult to know whether or not this is due to cause and effect.

Case 11
A failure of antituberculous treatment

An Indian student presented at the age of 21 with a minor episode of haemoptysis. He gave a three-month history of weight loss from 63 kg to 55 kg, persistent cough for three months and a fever for two weeks. He was a haemophiliac from a family of haemophiliac males. He was admitted to hospital and given factor VIII to control the haemoptysis. Sputum was positive for mycobacterium tuberculosis on direct smear. The initial chest radiograph had shown right apical shadowing with cavitation (**1**). Isoniazid, rifampicin and pyrazinamide were commenced. Following four months of outpatient treatment, there had been no improvement in his condition and no weight increase, and night sweating continued. The chest radiograph showed some improvement, but a large cavity was now present (**2**). As the patient had become jaundiced, his medication was changed to isoniazid, ethambutol and thiacetazone. He was found to be hepatitis B-positive. He began to develop sickness, and seemed reluctant to take his medication as he felt this was directly causing his symptoms. Sputum continued to be positive on smear and culture for acid- and alcohol-fast bacilli (AAFB). The isoniazid was stopped, and he continued on ethambutol and thiacetazone. He became rather violent towards his medical carer and refused to take some of his medication. Over the next year he continued on a chronic course, taking intermittent medication and without any overall improvement in symptomatology, weight gain or in the chest radiographic appearances (**3**). A CT scan three years after initial presentation showed extensive right upper-lobe disease (**4**). A sputum sample taken four years after his initial presentation was positive on direct smear and culture. Sensitivity results showed him to be resistant to isoniazid, streptomycin, kanamycin and pyrazinamide, but sensitive to ethambutol, rifampicin and cycloserin. He was started on rifampicin, cycloserin and pyrazinamide, and was maintained on a course of ethambutol, cycloserin and ciprofloxacin; however, he continued to have intermittent haemoptysis requiring factor VIII.

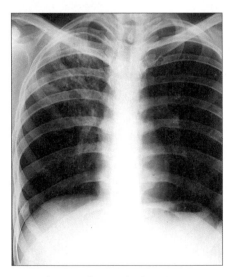

1 PA chest radiograph showing characteristic soft shadowing at right apex and mid zone.

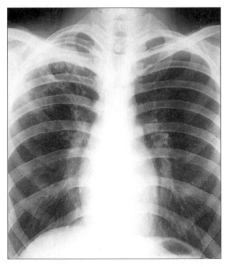

2 PA chest radiograph after four months of treatment showing considerable clearance, but a large cavity remains in the periphery of the right upper zone.

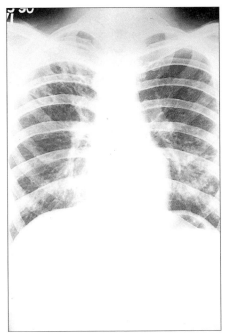

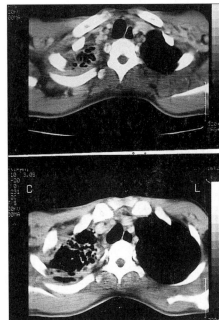

3 PA chest radiograph one year after **2** showing widespread shadowing at right apex.

4 Two cuts of a CT scan taken shortly after **3** showing collapse, consolidation and cavitation in the right apex.

QUESTIONS
1. What factors contributed to the patient's drug resistance?
2. What measures might have been taken to avoid its development?
3. What principles of treatment should be used in the presence of drug resistance?

Case 11

1. This somewhat tragic case demonstrates the poor prognosis of a multiple drug-resistant tuberculosis. Although the individual was a haemophiliac, repeated tests for human immunodeficiency virus (HIV) were negative. The hepatic complications no doubt added to the overall debility of the patient, and may have been contributed to his lack of response to a regimen to which the bacteria were initially sensitive on *in vitro* testing. Added hepatic complications also prevented the use of rifampicin, although this was introduced later when the patient's condition became critical. The reasons for drug resistance emerging in a patient who initially had fully drug-sensitive organisms is usually due to the patient's response to the regimen; in this case, he at times became aggressive towards his medical carer, and it is therefore likely that he abused the drug regimen he was given. As a side-effect of isoniazid is psychosis, the drug should have been stopped initially and then restarted cautiously to determine whether this was the case.
2. Combined chemotherapy with several antibiotics contained in a single tablet was not available in his country of treatment, so this means of prevention of emergence of multiple drug resistance was not available to his medical practitioners. However, management might have been improved by continuous in-patient treatment with fully supervised therapy at the start of the illness.
3. A) In the presence of drug resistance, patients should be given at least two anti-tuberculous drugs which they have not received previously.
   B) Never add a single drug to a failing regimen.

Further History

This patient did not respond to the second-line drug regimes, and continued to deteriorate clinically and radiographically (**5**). He developed increasing shadowing in the right upper lobe, and the cavity eventually contained a mycetoma (**6**). He died of liver complications some five years after presentation.

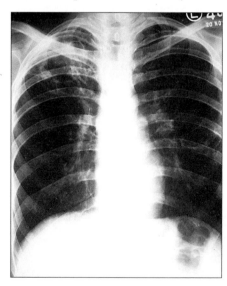 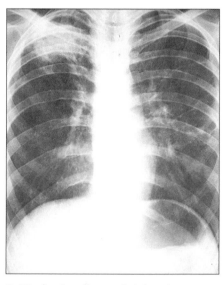

5 PA chest radiograph taken one year after **4**, showing extensive cavitation in the right apex.

6 PA chest radiograph taken two months after **5**, showing opacification of a cavity, probably from a mycetoma.

Case 12
Double diagnosis

A Chinese man aged 62 years presented with a two-month history of pain in the right arm, with numbness in the tips of the fingers. He had had a smoker's cough for many years, having smoked 20 cigarettes a day since a teenager, but had had no haemoptysis. There was no family history of tuberculosis. He had been living in the United Kingdom for 36 years since emigrating from Hong Kong. He had undergone partial gastrectomy and cholecystectomy many years previously. He suffered from maturity onset diabetes and was taking diclofenic sodium, gliclazide and co-proxamol. He lived with his wife and sons, and tended to drink heavily; however, he said he had not drunk alcohol for the previous two months. On examination, he had obvious pain in the right arm, but there were no abnormal signs in the chest, cardiovascular system or abdomen. Due to his poor English, a neurological examination was difficult, but he appeared to have diminished sensation in his fingers. The chest radiograph is shown in **1**. He underwent a bronchoscopy and bronchial lavage. the bronchoscopy was normal and he was subsequently started on tablets. Three weeks after he had been started on treatment, he presented with increasing pain in the right arm and shoulder. The radiograph of the upper right humerus is shown in **2**.

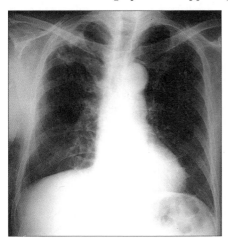

1 PA chest radiograph.

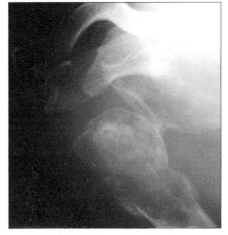

2 Radiograph of right humerus.

Investigations

Haemoglobin (Hb):	11.7 g/dl
WBC:	9.1×10^9/L (76.8% lymph; 13.0% neutrophils)
Erythrocyte sedimentation rate (ESR):	90 mm in the first hour
Calcium:	2.38 (2.18–2.61) mmol/L
Albumin:	39 (35–50) g/L
Alkaline phosphatase:	247 (30–130) IU/L

QUESTIONS
1. What diagnosis would you consider?
2. What are the causes of the appearances in **2**, and how would you confirm the diagnosis?
3. What further management would you consider?

Case 12

1. A cavitating chest lesion is most likely to be either a carcinoma or tuberculosis. The smear of the bronchial lavage fluid (**3**) shows typical and acid-fast bacilli of tuberculosis. Hence, he was started on antituberculous chemotherapy.

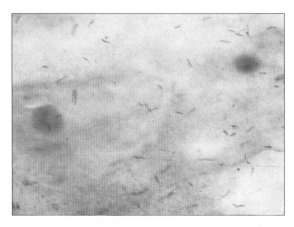

3 Sputum smear.

2. There is a fracture with bony obstruction of the humerus. The possible causes include simple trauma due to secondary carcinoma. Tuberculosis can present at a bony site, usually in the presence of disease in the lungs. When presenting in bone, tuberculosis usually causes insidious abscess and sinus formation which may be painful. Presentation as a fracture is extremely rare. Biopsy of the fracture site is the only method of establishing the diagnosis.

3. The histology of the fracture site showed a squamous-cell carcinoma (**4**).

   The lesion was assumed to be a secondary lesion from the lung primary. Had the bone lesion been due to tuberculosis, conservative therapy with continuing anti-tuberculous chemotherapy and immobilisation of the fracture site would have been sufficient. Lung carcinoma occurs in 2–5% of patients with pulmonary tuberculosis, usually in elderly patients with a smoking history. It is probable that the carcinoma develops first, causing a local immunodeficiency which allows tuberculosis infection to develop into overt disease.

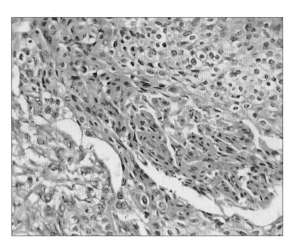

4 A section of biopsy from the fracture site, showing squamous-cell carcinoma.

Case 13
An acute illness in a young girl

A 16-year-old girl with a past history of well-controlled bronchial asthma developed a dry cough and sore throat and was thought to be suffering from the common cold. Three days later when her unproductive cough was more troublesome, she complained of a sharp, right-sided chest pain and developed a fever of 38.4°C. She was given paracetamol but her fever continued and the right-sided chest pain made breathing painful. She complained of soreness in her mouth and was started on amoxycillin 250 mg three times daily.

Twenty-four hours later her condition deteriorated and she was admitted to hospital. She had a productive cough, and on examination looked 'toxic'. Her temperature was 39°C, her blood pressure was 120/70 mmHg, and she had a rash around and in her mouth (1). Her breathing was rapid and shallow (respiratory rate 25 per minute), and examination of the chest revealed that the trachea was central with a reduced percussion note at the right lung base. On auscultation there was reduced air entry over the right lower lobe, together with some fine inspiratory crackles and abnormal breath sounds. The chest radiograph was abnormal (2).

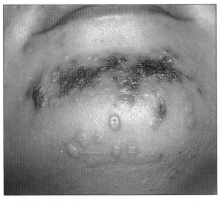

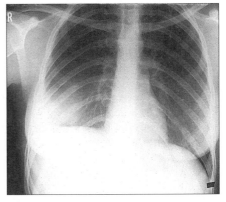

1 Rash around and in patient's mouth.   **2** Chest radiograph with abnormalities.

Investigations

Haematology:	Hb:	1.2 g/dl
	WBC:	15.1×10^9/L (90% neutrophils)
Biochemistry:	Serum sodium:	126 mmol/L
	Potassium :	3.6 mmol/L
	Urea:	3.7 mmol/L
Blood gases:	pH:	7.4
	PaO_2:	8.7 kPa
	$PaCO_2$:	3.8 kPa

QUESTIONS
1. What does **1** show?
2. Describe the abnormalities in the radiograph (**2**). What abnormal breath sounds would you expect to hear? Explain why they occur.
3. What is the likely diagnosis? List the common causes.
4. What other investigation(s) would you arrange?

Case 13

1. **1** shows 'cold sores' due to type 1 herpes simplex viral infection. After a primary infection (usually in childhood), the virus is thought to remain latent in the sensory ganglia of the trigeminal nerve. Reactivation occurs with a variety of stimuli, of which the most common is, as in this case, a rise in temperature from any cause.

2. The chest radiograph (**2**) showed shadowing at the right lung base, suggesting consolidation, and the abnormal lung sounds were bronchial breathing. This occurs when sounds from patent central airways pass through consolidated lung. Normal lungs filter out high-frequency sounds, but when consolidated these high-frequency sounds travel to the chest wall, producing the phenomenon of bronchial breathing.

3. The diagnosis is of community-acquired pneumonia. In up to 75% of cases, the infective organism is *Streptococcus pneumoniae*. The main alternative in this case is *Mycoplasma pneumoniae*, which commonly occurs in young people.

4. The investigations are directed towards isolating the infective organism and assessing the severity of the pneumonia:

   a) Detection of the organism: in all cases, patients should, if possible, have sputum sent for culture and sensitivities. However, in up to one third of cases, patients do not expectorate, and physiotherapy, saline nebulisation and even invasive techniques such as bronchoscopy may be appropriate in severe cases. The results of sputum tests must be interpreted with caution, as they may contain organisms from the upper respiratory tract. Blood cultures should always be taken. In this case, the blood cultures were positive for *S. pneumoniae*. **3** shows a typical morphology of *S. pneumoniae*.

   b) Viruses *Coxiella burnetti*, *Mycoplasma pneumoniae* and *Legionella* spp. are not easy to culture, and results of serology have to be used in most cases. Thus it is wise to send an initial sera on admission to hospital, but the results of rising antibody titres (four-fold increase) may not be seen early enough to be of use in the initial management of the patient. A single high titre is, however, a useful indication of the organism involved, and for *Mycoplasma* a high titre of specific immunoglobulin M is usually present. Recently, antigen tests in serum and urine, particularly for pneumococci, are available, providing a rapid test for the presence of specific infections.

   c) Assessment of severity: the three most important discriminating factors for disease severity are a respiratory rate of 30 per minute, a diastolic blood pressure of 60 mmHg or less and a serum urea above 7 mmol/L. When two or more of these are positive, there is usually a need for intensive care management.

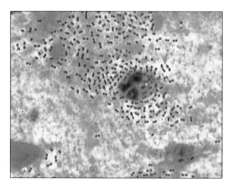

3 Typical morphology of *Streptococcus pneumoniae*. (Courtesy of Dr. M. E. Hodson. Reprinted from Turner-Warwick, Hodson, Corrin and Kerr, *Clinical Atlas of Respiratory Diseases*, 1989, Gower Medical Publishing.)

Further history

Following the initial treatment, the patient's temperature settled, but within two days she developed a swinging fever (4). The chest radiograph at this time is also seen (5).

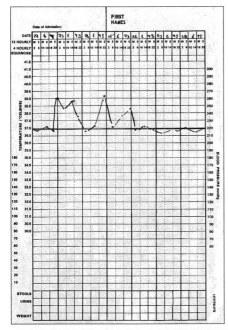

4 Temperature chart showing patient's swinging fever.

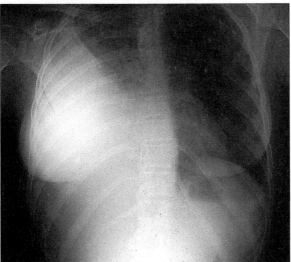

5 Chest radiograph.

QUESTIONS

1. What treatment would you have initiated when this patient arrived at hospital?
2. What complication has occurred to cause the treatment to fail?
3. How would you investigate and manage this complication?

Case 13

ANSWERS

1. The correct treatment depends on the initial assessment of the pneumonia. In this case, she was not ill enough to need intensive care treatment, but there was moderate hypoxaemia, requiring supplemental oxygen of 35%. She was given intravenous antibiotics for the first 48 hours to cover the common pathogenic organisms (particularly *S. pneumoniae*), initially amoxycillin 500 mg tds (her previous oral dosage was too low). Because she was young and there was a possibility of *Mycoplasma* infection, erythromycin was also added but was discontinued 24 hours later when *S. pneumoniae* was grown from the blood cultures.

2. The chest radiograph (**5**) shows a large pleural effusion. When this is associated with a swinging fever, the possibility of an empyema must be considered. **6** is a CT scan of this patient's thorax, showing the typical features of pleural fluid. CT scans can also be used to measure tissue density (Housefield number); in this case, the shadowing was caused by fluid density.

3. Whenever there is a pleural effusion associated with pneumonia, a pleural aspiration must be performed. In many cases this is a clear exudate; however, if it contains large numbers of leucocytes, an empyema may be developing. In this case, offensive-smelling creamy pus was aspirated, confirming the presence of an empyema.

   The most widely accepted management of an empyema is to drain it with a large intercostal drainage tube (e.g. 32-inch french gauge tube) inserted into the lower part of the empyema. However, the correct placement of the tube can be difficult. If there is a problem, the use of chest ultrasound can be helpful. **7** shows a typical ultrasound trace, demonstrating the presence of fluid. Care must be taken when inserting a tube between the lower ribs, as the liver or spleen can be damaged. As a general rule, a tube must never be inserted if pus cannot be obtained by simple needle aspiration. The drain must be attached to an underwater seal. Antibiotic cover has to be prolonged, and it is usual to include metronidazole to cover anaerobic infections, particularly if the fluid is foul smelling (as was the case in this patient).

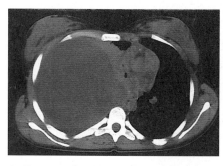

6 CT scan of patient's thorax showing typical features of pleural fluid.

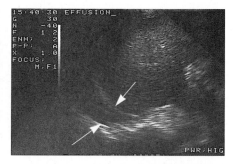

7 Typical ultrasound trace demonstrating presence of fluid (*arrowed*).

Further history

After draining the empyema, the patient's temperature settled. However, two weeks later her temperature suddenly became elevated again. A chest radiograph at the time was satisfactory, and no abnormal physical signs were elicited.

QUESTIONS
1. How long would you leave the intercostal drainage tube *in situ*?
2. Give at least two possible reasons why this patient's temperature became elevated for a second time.
3. What are the long-term sequelae of empyemas?

ANSWERS
1. The intercostal tube is left *in situ* until the empyema has completely cleared. Problems with loculation of the empyema pus are common, and may require a second tube. Care must be taken to prevent the drain(s) from becoming dislodged and falling out of the chest. If drainage is not complete after two weeks, a surgical opinion needs to be sought, as debridement of the empyema space may be required.
2. There are many possibilities for the late rise in temperature. This could be due to loculated pus in the chest but this was not seen on the chest radiograph. Metastatic abscesses can occur in other organs, particularly if the empyema is due to *Streptococcus milleri*. However, in this case, shortly after the development of the fever, a generalised maculo-papular rash occurred (**8**). This is typical of antibiotic allergy, and thus the likely diagnosis was a penicillin drug fever. After changing to erythromycin, the temperature settled and the patient made an uneventful recovery.
3. The most common long-term sequelae of empyema is pleural thickening. A thick, fibrous 'peel' can encase the lung and diminish movement of the affected hemithorax, with a restrictive ventilatory defect. Treatment is with surgical decortication. Occasionally an empyema becomes chronic, and may discharge though a sinus over many years. Fortunately, with modern treatment this is now very rare.

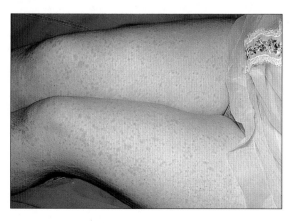

8 Generalised maculo-papular rash developing after fever.

Case 14

Painful arthropathy

Over a period of two months, a 63-year-old man complained of painful wrists and ankles which were becoming progressively more painful, and his sleep had become disturbed. When seen by his general practitioner, he looked well and there was no obvious swelling around the wrists or ankles, but there was marked local tenderness and the joints felt hot to the touch. A photograph of his hand is seen in **1**. An abnormality was also seen when examining his chest, as seen in **2**.

The patient's only previous illness was duodenal ulceration for which he had cholecystectomy. He gave up cigarette smoking three years ago, but between the age of 16 and 60 he had consumed an average of 10 cigarettes per day. Throughout his working life he had been a clerical worker, and very rarely needed time off work.

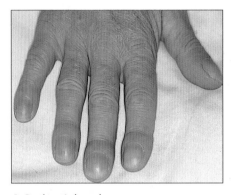

1 Patient's hand.

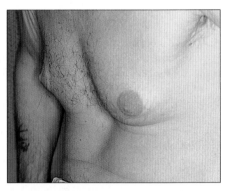

2 Abnormality in patient's chest.

Investigations

Initial biochemical investigations were all normal.	
Hb:	11.2 g/dl
WBC:	8.5×10^9/L
ESR:	88 mm in the first hour
FEV_1:	1.6 L (3.2)
FVC:	2.5 L (4.2)
FEV_1:	65%
Rheumatoid factor:	Negative.
Antinuclear antibody:	Negative.
Radiology:	Radiograph of hands and wrists (**3** and **4**)
	Bone scan of wrist (**5**) and ankles (**6**)

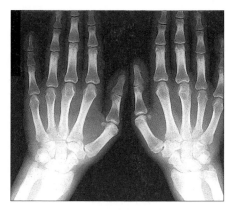

3 Radiograph of hands and wrists.

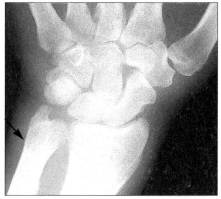

4 Close-up of wrist with abnormality (*arrowed*).

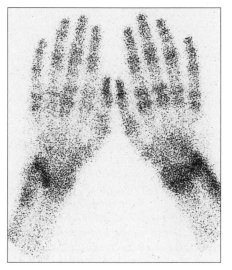

5 Bone scan of hands and wrists.

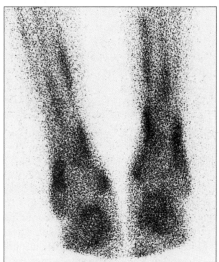

6 Bone scan of ankles.

QUESTIONS

1. What does the photograph of the hand show? List six causes.
2. What does the radiograph of the hand and wrist (**3** and **4**) show? Relate this to the isotope bone scan (**5**) and clinical symptoms. What is the cause of this condition?
3. What is the abnormality seen on the photograph of the chest (**2**)? List the common causes.
4. What do you think is the most likely diagnosis in this patient? Outline what further investigations you would perform.
5. How would you estimate this patient's total exposure to cigarettes?
6. What initial treatment would you give, and what other treatment may help this condition?

Case 14

1. The photograph of this patient's hands show marked finger clubbing associated with 'drumstick' deformity of the fingertips. Clubbing occurs most commonly in respiratory diseases, particularly carcinoma of the bronchus, suppurative conditions (e.g. bronchiectasis, empyema or abscess), and diffuse interstitial fibrosis (e.g. cryptogenic fibrosing alveolitis, asbestosis and sarcoidosis); however, it is much less common in extrinsic allergic alveolitis. Cardiac causes include untreated subacute bacterial endocarditis and cyanotic heart disease. Clubbing is also seen in hepatic cirrhosis and ulcerative colitis, and on occasions may be inherited as a benign familial condition.

2. When there is marked finger clubbing, patients may complain of arthritis of the wrists and ankles with local tenderness. On palpation, the joints and surrounding tissue feel hot. This condition is known as hypertrophic pulmonary osteo-arthropathy (HPOA). The diagnosis is confirmed by a radiograph of the wrist that shows a periosteal reaction with new bone formation as indicated in **4**. The bone scan shows increased uptake of the isotope in the distal long bones associated with the marked periosteal activity. The cause of clubbing and HPOA is not known, but is probably mediated by a marked increase in the periosteal blood flow. This may be mediated by substances secreted by some tumour tissues, since after resection the clubbing and HPOA may disappear. HPOA has been reported with other tumours and lymphomas, and also with chronic suppurative conditions.

3. **2** shows gynaecomastia, which in the adult is always pathological. As with this patient, the breasts are often painful. Causes include: drugs (e.g. digoxin and spironolactone); excess circulating oestrogens as in hepatic failure; oestrogen treatment for prostatic carcinoma; or oestrogen-like compounds secreted by tumours, particularly squamous carcinoma of the bronchus.

4. The most likely diagnosis to account for this patient's symptoms, physical signs and investigations is a bronchial neoplasm. A chest radiograph (**7**) confirms the presence of a tumour in the right lung. A fibre-optic bronchoscopy confirmed tumour in the bronchus intermedius, and a biopsy sent for histology confirmed the presence of a squamous-cell carcinoma. A CT scan was performed to ascertain if there was local lymphatic mediastinal spread and to look for a tumour in common secondary sites, particularly the liver (**8**) and adrenal glands. Unfortunately, the scan confirmed metastasis in both the mediastinal glands and liver.

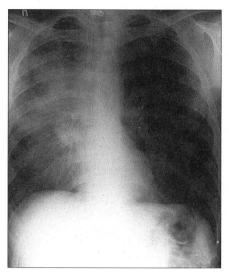

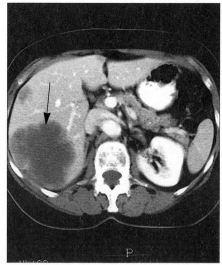

7 Chest radiograph showing a tumour in the right lung.

8 CT scan of liver with metastases (*arrowed*).

5. This patient had smoked cigarettes from the age of 16 to 60, a total smoking history of 44 years. It is usual to estimate smoking in pack years (one pack year being 20 cigarettes per day for one year). In this case, 10 cigarettes per day for a year is half a pack year, therefore his total exposure was 22 pack years. However, caution is necessary as patients often underestimate their cigarette consumption.

6. The initial treatment was to try and alleviate the distressing symptoms of HPOA. A non-steroidal analgesic provided some relief, as did a small dose of prednisolone. Vagotomy has also been suggested as a treatment. HPOA is known to respond to the removal of the primary site, but in this case the tumour was inoperable. Thus, the only other possibilities were chemotherapy or radiotherapy. Radiotherapy was the preferred option; however, the HPOA symptoms remained troublesome, and this necessitated the use of narcotic analgesics in the form of twice-daily sustained-release morphine sulphate.

Case 15
Complications after surgery

A 70-year-old man noticed weakness and parasthesia of his hands and progressive difficulty in walking. On examination, he was found to have wasting of the small muscles of his hands and upper motor neurone signs in his legs. A radiograph of his cervical spine showed extensive changes of cervical spondylosis, and a diagnosis of cervical myelopathy was made. A magnetic resonance scan (1) confirmed compression of the cervical cord at C3/5 and C4/5 levels.

The spinal cord was decompressed by an anterior cervical microdiscectomy, and post-operatively there was evidence of some improvement of his neurological signs. On the third post-operative day, he developed a cough productive of purulent sputum and a fever of 37.5°C. The chest radiograph did not show any inflammatory changes, but he was started on a course of oral amoxicillin at 500 mg three times daily. His temperature settled, but ten days later his condition deteriorated. He was again pyrexial, with a swinging temperature of up to 39°C; he expectorated up to half a cup full of purulent sputum daily and became a little confused. On examination, he looked cyanosed, and there was reduced percussion over the right anterior chest wall; coarse inspiratory crackles were heard over the same area on ausculation. The following investigations were performed:

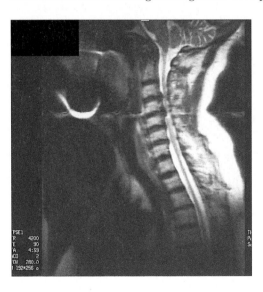

1 Magnetic resonance image (MRI) of cervical cord.

Investigations

Hb:	11.6 g/dl
WBC:	25.9×10^9/L (91 % neutrophils)
pH:	7.4
PaO_2:	7.4 kPa
$PaCO_2$:	4.9 kPa
Radiology:	Chest radiograph (2)
	CT scan of right upper lobe (3)
Blood cultures:	No growth
Sputum cytology:	(see 4)
Sputum culture of *Pseudomonas aeruginosa*	

2 Chest radiograph.

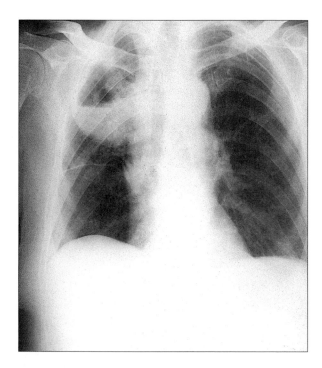

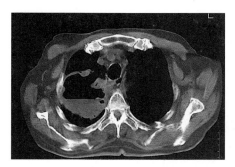

3 CT scan of right upper lobe.

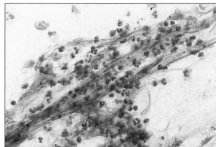

4 Sputum cytology.

QUESTIONS

1. What abnormality is seen on the chest radiograph and CT scan?
2. List the differential diagnoses, and state which are the two most common causes.
3. What is the most likely diagnosis (listing your reasons), and the underlying aetiology?
4. What would you have expected from sputum cultures?
5. What other investigation(s) would you arrange?
6. What treatments would you initiate, and how long would you continue these treatments?
7. What complications may occur?

Case 15

1. The chest radiograph shows a large cavitating lesion in the right upper lobe. This is confirmed on the CT scan, and on this image the presence of fluid in the cavity is easily seen. This was found to vary with posture.
2. The differential diagnosis of a cavitating chest lesion is listed in **Table 1**. The commonest causes are carcinoma of the bronchus and a simple infective lung abscess.

Table 1 Causes of fluid-filled cavities on a chest radiograph

- Lung abscess
- Encysted empyema
- Cavitating tumour (particularly squamous-cell carcinoma)
- Infected bulla or bronchial cyst
- Wegener's granulomatosis
- Hydatid cyst
- Cavitating rheumatoid nodule
- Infected pulmonary infarction
- Gas-fluid level in intrathoracic oesophagus, stomach or bowel

3. In this case, the history, presence of fever, high white-cell count, expectoration of large quantities of purulent sputum (**5**) and the chest radiograph are characteristic of an infective lung abscess. It was almost certainly caused by aspiration from the oropharynx during or just after the patient's surgery. It is quite common for the abscess to develop over a period of two or three weeks.

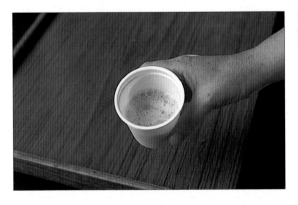

5 Purulent sputum—this cup was filled in 24 hours.

4. The organisms found in the sputum of patients with lung abscess are most commonly anaerobic, and these can be difficult to culture. However, they often impart a characteristically foul smell to the sputum. In this case, *Pseudomonas aeruginosa* was the only pathogen isolated, but it is likely that other organisms such as *Bacteroides* spp. were also present. Failure to isolate any organism from the sputum is not uncommon, in which case tracheal or bronchoscopic specimens can be helpful.

5. It is wise to perform a bronchoscopy to exclude a tumour or foreign body and to obtain material for microbiology. In this case, the bronchoscopy showed no endobronchial lesion, but large quantities of purulent material were coming from the right upper lobe.

6. Appropriate antibiotic treatment is very important. As *Pseudomonas aeruginosa* was cultured, intravenous ceftazidine was used for 10 days, followed by oral ciprofloxacin. In addition, because of the possibility of a mixed culture of anaerobic organisms, oral metronidazole was added. Antibiotic treatment should normally be continued for six weeks. Physiotherapy and postural drainage helps to drain the pus from the bronchial tree. In those cases where drainage does not occur, intervention to establish drainage is now being advocated. This can be achieved either endobronchially at bronchoscopy or percutaneously. Occasional abscesses which do not respond to treatment have to be resected surgically.

7. In the pre-antibiotic era, progression of a lung abscess to an empyema was common, and occasionally, a metastatic abscess developed. The erosion of blood vessels within the cavity may result in haemoptysis, which can be life-threatening. Longer-term complications include bronchiectasis and the development of an aspergilloma. All the usual complications of immobility may occur, and in this patient an extensive deep-vein thrombosis developed, confirmed on a venogram. He was anticoagulated, but afterwards developed a gastrointestinal haemorrhage. Despite this he subsequently made a full recovery. A radiograph taken six weeks after the onset of his illness is seen (**6**), showing almost complete resolution of the abscess cavity.

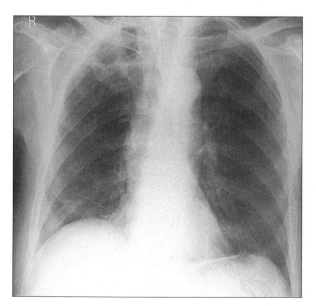

6 Chest radiograph.

A man with increasing breathlessness of recent onset

A previously fit 47-year-old man presents with a history of increasing breathlessness on exertion and in the evenings over the past six months. His symptoms did not occur every day, but when they did he noticed that they tended to be worse in the early evening after he returned home from work, and the symptoms would generally ease off by the time he went to bed. He described feeling tight-chested, but did not think he wheezed. He had also noticed having difficulty keeping up with his wife while walking on level ground, because his chest felt tight and he was coughing. He occasionally woke up at nights with marked breathlessness, such that he had to get up and make himself a cup of tea. The symptoms had subsided over an hour or two.

Ten years earlier, he developed a smoker's cough, and on advice stopped smoking. His father had died of lung cancer, but there was no family history of asthma or atopy. He had kept a pet dog for the last four years. For the last 10 years he had been employed on the docks as a labourer, and prior to that had been a council dustbin man for 20 years. He rarely had time off work, but in the last six months had had three periods of illness, the first lasting two weeks, the second, three weeks and the third for 10 weeks. He was still off work and his job was now at risk. On examination he appeared well, was of good colour and was not distressed at rest.

There were no abnormalities of the heart or respiratory system. The chest radiograph and ECG were normal, and his spirometry showed an FEV_1 of 3.6 L (97% predicted) and an FVC of 4.8 L, giving a FEV_1/FVC ratio of 75. His peak flow at the clinic was 510 L/min. Routine blood samples revealed a normal blood count, normal biochemistry and an IgE of 126 IU/L. His general practitioner had given him a peak-flow meter (1) a few weeks earlier and had asked him to record a peak-flow chart, which he then showed to the doctor (2). A histamine challenge test (3 and 4) showed that he had significantly increased bronchial hyper-reactivity (concentration provoking a 20% fall in FEV_1 [PC_{20}] was 0.025 mg/ml).

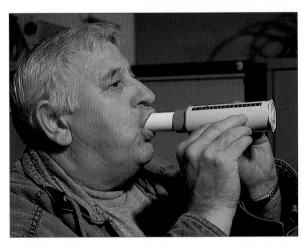

1 A peak-flow meter in use. It is easy to use, portable and cheap. Single values are of limited value but serial measurements are highly diagnostic.

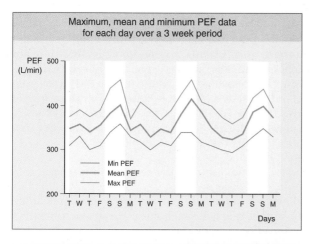

2 Serial PEF values over three weeks at home and at work. (Shaded areas represent times when the patient was at work.)

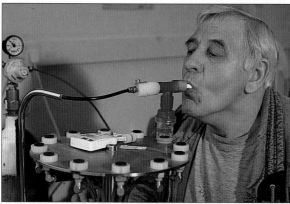

3 Histamine challenge test being performed. Subjects inhale doubling concentrations of histamine until their FEV$_1$ falls by 20%.

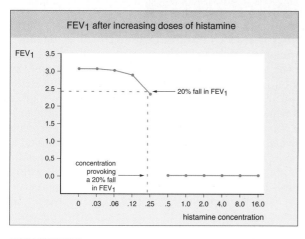

4 Chart of lung function FEV$_1$ against increasing dose of histamine.

QUESTIONS

1. What questions would you ask this man to elucidate the cause of his symptoms?
2. How would you go about investigating his troubles, and what advice would you give him?

Case 16

1. The history is suggestive of late-onset asthma. Chest tightness and cough are common presenting symptoms, and patients may be unaware that they are wheezing. The exertional chest tightness could be exercise asthma or could be due to ischaemic heart disease. The peak-flow chart shows that his PEF varies from under 300 L to over 500 L/min when seen at clinic, which is highly suggestive of asthma. The chart also shows that the mean PEF was 350 L/min while at work, rising to over 400 L while at home during the weekend. This is suggestive, but not diagnostic, of a work relationship. The questions to be asked are:

   A. What was he handling at his work?

   B. Were his symptoms better when off work at the weekend or when on holiday?

   He responded that for the past four years he had been working on unloading grain from the holds of ships and storing it in warehouses. The job was often very dusty (**5**), and although masks had been provided he often took them off because they were uncomfortably hot. He did not handle grain every day, but thought on reflection that it could have been on those days that his chest was worse in the evenings.

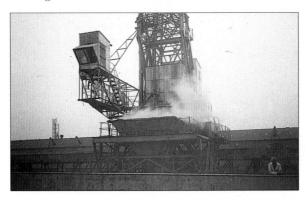

5 During unloading of grain, clouds of dust could envelop the workers.

2. The management problem is first to confirm asthma and then to establish whether it is the result of his job or unrelated late-onset asthma. Although he is now off work and has normal lung function, asthma can be confirmed by provoking airways obstruction using a histamine challenge test (as in this case) and/or an asthma exercise test (six minutes' exercise followed by a peak expiratory flow [PEF] recording for 15 minutes). Histamine bronchial hyper-reactivity is sensitive but not specific, whereas the airways obstruction after exercise is specific, but is only positive in about 70% of asthmatics. Since his livelihood is at stake, the relationship to work must be established positively, which usually means returning to work while continuing to record PEF charts, but recording values much more frequently—every two hours—in order to be able to appreciate changes occurring within the day and the temporal relationship to exposures. In this man's case, as he was reluctant to return to work, a specific challenge test was recorded in the laboratory which consisted of exposure either to a placebo (lactose powder) or to some of the grain dust collected from his workplace for one hour each on different days in a challenge chamber (**6**). This showed that he had no early response, but beginning at five hours developed significant wheeze and airflow limitation only to the grain dust (**7**).

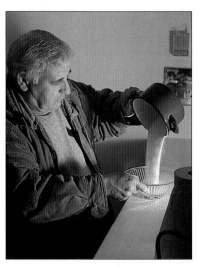

6 Exposure to test dust within a challenge chamber, which ensures that only the subject and not the technician is exposed.

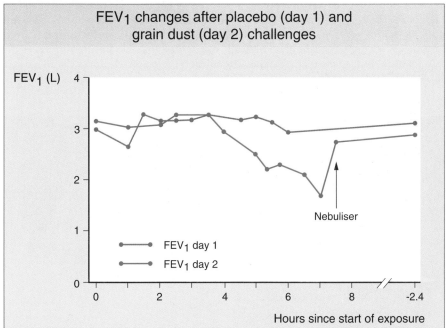

7 Results of challenge testing showing a 26% fall in FEV_1 at five hours after exposure to the grain dust, but no response to a lactose placebo.

This late-phase response explains his initial description of evening symptoms and is well described in grain worker's asthma, although it is not true for the majority of occupational asthma cases who will have an early (15–30-minute response) and thus are often easier to diagnose.

Since ceasing work this man's symptoms have been much better, although he remains prone to cough and tight-chestedness when he has a cold.

Case 17
A water-logged patient

A 66-year-old man with a temperature and worsening breathlessness was sent by his general practitioner to the casualty ward (**1**). He was cyanosed and was breathless when at rest, with an easily audible expiratory wheeze. His wife explained that he had been chesty for many years, with episodes of chesty bronchitis most winters that had been treated at home with courses of antibiotics. He had not worked for over ten years, having lost his job as a building site labourer because he was too breathless to climb ladders. He had smoked heavily (more than 30 cigarettes per day) until last winter when, during an exacerbation, he had suddenly decided to stop following a locum general practitioner's advice. Since then he had coughed less sputum, but had remained very breathless, so that he only went out of the house when his son collected him in the car. He and his wife lived in a bungalow, so he was able to manage for himself most of the time. However, he was occasionally unable to get to the toilet in time after taking his diuretic tablets (which he took to stop his ankles swelling). He had never been in hospital before. In the last week he had been too breathless to get out of bed, was coughing up dirty, greenish-coloured sputum, and the ankle swelling had not responded to the tablets. On examination, the doctor noted that the jugular venous pressure was raised (**2**) and was pulsatile; there was oedema of the legs reaching to the knees (**3**) and also some sacral oedema; and the patient's hands and feet were warm in spite of the cold winter temperatures. There were a few scattered coarse crackles and some generalised expiratory wheezes on auscultation, but no focal chest signs. The chest radiograph (**4**) and ECG (**5**) are as shown. His peak flow was 60 L/min.

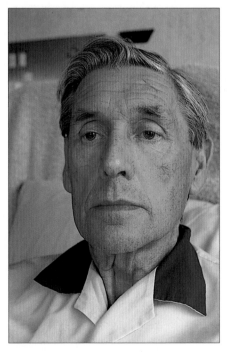

1 A 66-year-old breathless man.

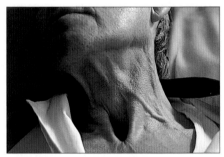

2 The jugular venous pulse.

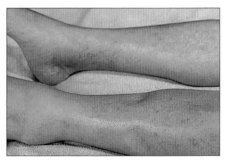

3 The ankles.

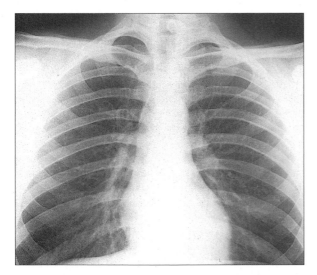

4 The PA chest radiograph.

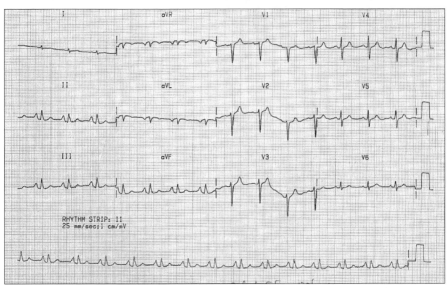

5 ECG.

QUESTIONS

1. What is your differential diagnosis? What is the first measurement you would make now?
2. What does the ECG show, and what are the changes due to? Are the changes permanent?
3. Does the chest radiograph help you in your diagnosis, and, if so, why?
4. What would this man's lung function tests show?
5. How would you treat him in A) the short term; and B) the long term?
6. If he were to deteriorate suddenly later that night, would you recommend intermittent positive pressure ventilation for him or not? Justify your decision.

Case 17

ANSWERS

1. This man has the signs of right heart failure with a raised jugular venous pressure and oedema. Sometimes congestive cardiac failure can present in this way, but the long history of winter bronchitis suggests that this is more likely to be cor pulmonale secondary to chronic obstructive pulmonary disease (COPD). The small heart size on the chest radiograph and the absence of any left heart strain on the ECG also favour a primary respiratory cause. COPD cannot be diagnosed confidently on clinical grounds alone, since primary alveolar hypoventilation and sleep apnoea syndromes can also lead to cor pulmonale, so it is always necessary to perform spirometry at some stage to confirm the diagnosis. The acute problem in this man is his cyanosis and breathlessness, so the first measurement should be a sample of arterial blood. In this man, the warm extremities should make you suspect that the CO_2 level will be raised. The actual values were pH 7.24, PaO_2 5.4 kPa and $PaCO_2$ 9.8 kPa, while the patient was already on a 24% oxygen mask. This man is therefore hypoventilating markedly (raised $PaCO_2$), leading to severe hypoxia. In addition, the low pH level shows that he has been retaining CO_2, particularly over the last few hours (the kidneys have not had time to compensate), so that there has been an acute deterioration which will need urgent treatment.

2. The ECG shows an axis shifted to the right (+105°) and a partial right-bundle branch-block pattern. In addition, the p waves are tall (>2 mm), representing a 'p' pulmonalae. These changes are the result of pulmonary hypertension, and will remain unless therapy (see below) is successful in reducing the level of pulmonary blood pressure. In many patients the changes will persist.

3. The chest radiograph is helpful in that it demonstrates a normal heart size and excludes severe left heart failure. It also shows no focal lung disease (tumour or lobar pneumonia), but it does not exclude the presence of some infection in the chest. The radiologists often report the irregular markings on this radiograph as indicating a 'chronic bronchitic' chest, but in fact there are no clinical studies to justify that these markings have any such implication. COPD must be diagnosed physiologically, not radiologically.

4. His lung function tests after the acute episode (*see* **Table 1**) showed that he has indeed got severe airways obstruction with a raised residual volume (RV) and a relatively preserved diffusing capacity ($D_L co$). After nebulised salbutamol, there was a small but non-significant change in his lung function, and after two weeks of oral steroids, the values were unchanged. His airflow obstruction is non-reversible.

Table 1 Lung function tests

	Actual	Predicted
FEV_1:	0.65 L	2.4 L
FEV_1 (after nebuliser)::	0.70 L	
FEV_1 (after oral steroids):	0.65 L	
FVC:	2.1 L	3.3 L
Residual volume:	3.1 L	1.8 L
Total lung capacity:	5.2 L	5.1 L
$D_L co$:	23.6 mm/min/mmHg	24.1 mm/min/mmHg

QMUL Library
Whitechapel Libray
Email: library@qmul.ac.uk
Tel: 020 7882 8800

Renew items, check loans and holds,
pay fines and more online at:

www.library.qmul.ac.uk/self_service

Borrowed Items 19/05/2014 09:20
XXXXXX245X

Item Title	Due Date
* Respiratory physiology : th	16/06/2014
* Key topics in respiratory m	27/05/2014
* ABC of COPD	27/05/2014
* ABC of asthma	16/06/2014
* Pulmonary physiology and	16/06/2014
* Pulmonary pathophysiolog	16/06/2014

Amount Outstanding : £0.80

---

* Indicates items borrowed today
Thank you for using
QMUL Whitechapel Library.

5. In the short term, this man needs to have his airways obstruction reversed as much as possible, and although the response to bronchodilators and/or to oral steroids may be very modest, both should be used. Small changes may result in significant improvements in the level of CO_2 retention. Antibiotics are needed to treat the presumed infection. In addition, a doxapram infusion can stimulate the level of resting ventilation and reduce the hypercapnia over the first 24–48 hours, thus 'buying time' for the other medications to take effect. The blood gases need to be repeated every few hours until it is clear that the pH and $PaCO_2$ are normalising.

In the longer term, this man is a potential candidate for long-term oxygen therapy (LTOT) at home (**6**) from a home oxygen concentrator (**7**). These devices use a molecular sieve to remove nitrogen from the air, leaving 95% oxygen at a flow of 2 L/min. Used 15 hours per day regularly, including throughout the night, LTOT can correct the most severe episodes of hypoxia, and thus reduce the tendency to develop pulmonary hypertension. Studies in Scotland and the US have shown that this can enhance both survival and quality of life as long as the hypoxia was definitely present and the patient had stopped smoking.

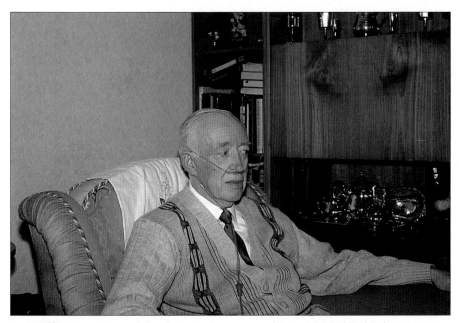

6 A different man receiving long-term oxygen therapy (LTOT) in his home.

Case 17

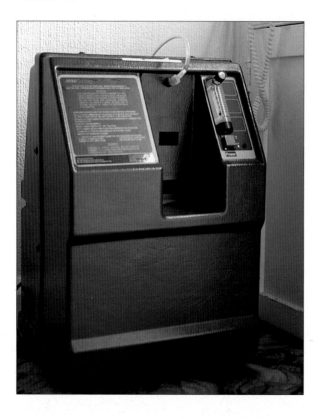

7 An oxygen concentrator installed in the home.

6. This is an extremely difficult question for which there is no simple universal answer, particularly as each case is different. However, there are some general principles which may help (**Table 2**).

Table 2

Likely to benefit:
- No previous admissions
- No previous documented history of chest disease
- Good performance status before this acute episode, e.g. able to get out to shops independently
- History suggestive of asthma
- Acute infection/empyema/lobar pneumonia

Likely not to benefit:
- Poor performance status before acute episode. e.g.. housebound or bedbound
- Concomitant diseases, e.g. rheumatoid arthritis or ischaemic heart disease
- * Extreme age (biological rather than chronological)
- Previous similar episodes in past year
- Well-documented severe and irreversible COPD (e.g. $FEV_1 < 0.6$ L)

Case 18
Congenital kyphoscoliosis

A 67-year-old man with a congenital kyphoscoliosis (**1**) was referred with a three-year history of progressively increasing dyspnoea and a two-year history of ankle swelling. Three years prior to presentation he had had an unlimited exercise tolerance, but on admission he was breathless after minimal exertion. He had no previous history of chest symptoms, and had not smoked for 20 years, but he had a total cigarette consumption of 30 pack years. Medication on admission was 40 mg of frusemide daily and an ipratropium bromide inhaler 40 µg four times daily.

On examination he had a gross kyphoscoliosis and was cyanosed. He had gross peripheral oedema to the mid-thoracic spine level. His jugular venous pressure (JVP) was elevated with prominent cannon waves, and auscultation of his heart revealed a pan-systolic murmur consistent with tricuspid regurgitation. Respiratory examination was unremarkable apart from a gross kyphoscoliosis.

Arterial blood gases taken while the patient was breathing air confirmed respiratory failure: PaO_2 4.7, $PaCO_2$ 7.91, pH 7.31.

An echocardiogram showed right ventricular hypertrophy and right atrial dilatation, with a poorly contracting right ventricle.

The chest radiograph (**2**) was difficult to interpret because of the gross kyphoscoliosis, but suggests cardiomegaly and a pleural effusion.

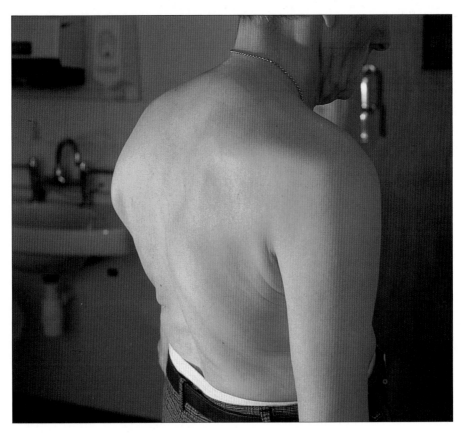

1 Patient showing kyphoscoliosis.

Case 18

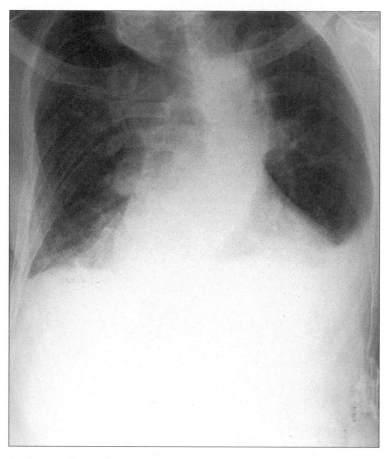

2 Chest radiograph.

IInvestigations

Baseline			Post-5 mg nebulised salbutamol		
	Predicted	**Measured**	**Predicted**	**Measured**	**Change**
FVC (l):	3.6 L	1.7	47%	1.79 L	5%
FEV_1 (l):	2.5 L	1.06	42%	1.03 L	-3%
FEV_1/FVC:		69%		62%	58%

	Measured	**Predicted**
Residual volume (RV):	1.66 L	73%
Functional residual capacity (FRC):	2.10 L	
Total lung capacity (TLC):	3.36 L	56%
Diffusing capacity ($D_L$co) :	11.7 ml/min/mmHg	50%

QUESTIONS

1. What is the likely cause of this gentleman's respiratory failure?
2. What do the ECG (**3**) and oximetry trace (**4**) show?
3. How would you manage this condition?
4. What is the prognosis?

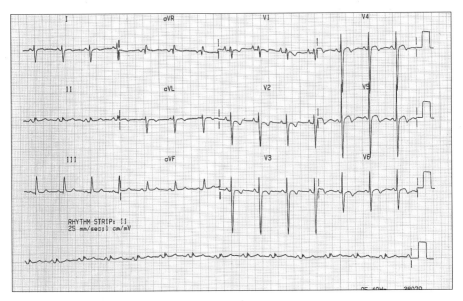

3 ECG.

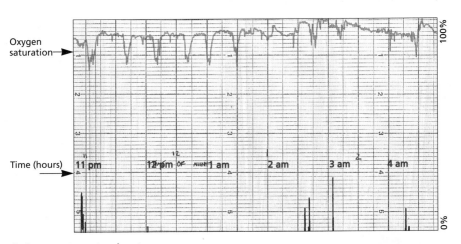

4 Pre-treatment oximetry.

Case 18

1. This gentleman's respiratory failure is secondary to his kyphoscoliosis. His previous cigarette consumption was quite modest, and he had not smoked for 20 years. This would make chronic obstructive pulmonary disease (COPD) unlikely. His pulmonary function tests show reduced lung volumes in contrast to the increased RV and FRC which would be expected in COPD. There was no change in his spirometry in response to nebulised bronchodilators, which is consistent with either 'irreversible' COPD or a restrictive chest wall problem.

    The sudden deterioration in his exercise tolerance from being previously unlimited is characteristic of patients with a thoracic cage deformity due to a kyphoscoliosis or a thoracoplasty performed many years previously as a treatment for tuberculosis in the pre-chemotherapy era.

2. The investigation of choice is a sleep study which measures oxygen saturation through the night. The illustration (4) shows simple overnight oximetry where oxygen saturation is continually recorded non-invasively by pulse oximetry. Periods of oxygen desaturation occur during rapid eye movement (REM) sleep (when skeletal muscle tone is at its minimum) with periods of normal oxygen saturation in between. As the condition progresses, the hypoxaemias present during other stages of sleep, and the patient may complain of morning headaches due to CO_2 retention. If untreated, the patient eventually develops persistent hypoxaemia even during the day, and consequently develops cor pulmonale. The ECG in 3 shows gross right ventricular hypertrophy. At the time of presentation, this gentleman's sleep studies showed persistent hypoxaemia with an oxygen saturation between 60% and 75% throughout the night.

3. The correct management of this condition depends on its recognition. His breathlessness and hypoxaemia had initially been ascribed to COPD; however, in chest wall deformity, bronchodilators are unhelpful (see the results of the spirometric reversibility tests). The correct treatment for a restrictive chest wall problem is non-invasive ventilatory support. This can be achieved either by positive pressure ventilation using a nasal mask or by negative pressure ventilation using a cuirass or tank ventilator. This patient was commenced on nocturnal nasal intermittent positive pressure ventilation (NIPPV) (5) and supplementary oxygen to maintain an oxygen saturation of around 90%. On this treatment and diuretic, his oedema settled and his exercise tolerance improved. At the time of discharge, his exercise tolerance had improved and he was able to walk around the ward without excessive dyspnoea. However, he remained hypoxic. He continued to use NIPPV at home, and his exercise tolerance and breathlessness improved steadily.

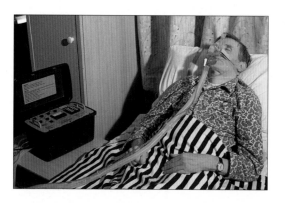

5 Oximetry on NIPPV.

4. The prognosis of respiratory failure secondary to a kyphoscoliosis is good, and the right ventricular hypertrophy and failure will regress. One year after discharge, this patient was reassessed in clinic. There was no evidence of ankle oedema, and his daytime gases showed PaO_2 8.2, $PaCO_2$ 5.2 and pH 7.33. His supplemental oxygen was withdrawn, and his diuretic treatment stopped. He remains well, with a six-minute walking distance of 240 m. Although he is able to maintain his oxygen saturation at rest, he desaturates quickly on modest exercise. **6** shows a graph of his oxygen saturation during a six-minute walking test, showing his desaturation from 93% to 85% within two minutes of starting the self-paced corridor walking test.

   Respiratory failure also occurs in other conditions where chest wall or diaphragmatic muscle function is impaired, as in the late stages of Duchenne and Charcot–Marie–Tooth muscular dystrophies and motor neurone disease. Non-invasive ventilation can be used effectively to palliate breathlessness and relieve distressing morning headaches due to CO_2 retention in these conditions. Likewise, assisted ventilation is the treatment of choice for the central sleep apnoea syndromes such as Ondine's curse.

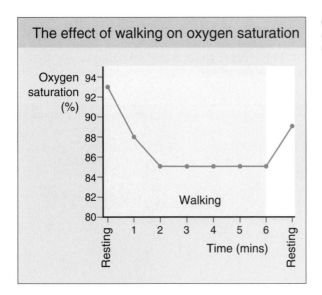

6 Graph of oxygen desaturation with exercise.

Case 19
A carpenter's tale

A 63 year-old-man presented with a history of breathlessness that had developed over the previous three weeks. He had not noticed any cough, sputum, haemoptysis or temperature, nor had he experienced any ankle swelling or central chest pain. However, he had noticed aching discomfort in his right side that responded to paracetamol, which was his only medication.

Prior to this illness, he had had a duodenal ulcer which was treated surgically when he was 35; he had had a slipped disc when he was 41, and a 'minor heart attack' when he was 45. Otherwise, he enjoyed good health, and had been working full-time as a carpenter. He smoked 20 cigarettes per day and had done so since the age of 15, and he drank 10–15 pints of beer over each weekend. His employment history included a seven-year period in the 1950s as a carpenter in the ship-building industry, and thereafter he had worked for the council's building department, helping to build and refurbish council houses.

On examination he was pink, breathed comfortably at rest but became mildly breathless while simply undressing. There was no finger clubbing; his blood pressure was 140/90 mmHg, but there were no signs of cardiac failure. The movement of his right chest was obviously limited, the percussion note was dull, and there was reduced air entry over the whole of the right hemithorax. There were no other clinical abnormalities. A pleural effusion was diagnosed (1), and the chest was aspirated to produce 1200 ml of straw-coloured fluid when drained. A pleural biopsy was taken (2), and because the fluid recurred within a week, formal drainage (3) and pleurodesis were performed. This relieved his breathlessness and eased his aching chest pain, but only temporarily. Six months later the chest radiograph looked worse (4).

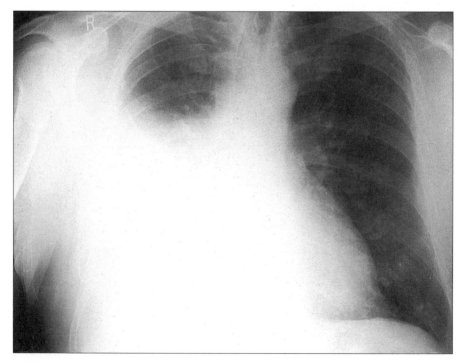

1 Chest radiograph on presentation.

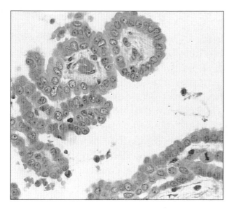

2 Pleural biopsy taken at the stage of the first radiograph.

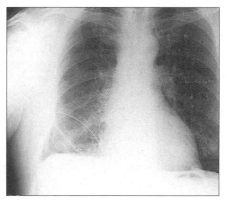

3 Chest radiograph with chest drain *in situ* showing almost complete radiological clearance.

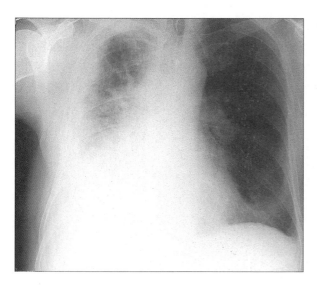

4 Chest radiograph six months later.

QUESTIONS

1. What laboratory results would you expect from the pleural fluid, and what do you see on the pleural biopsy?
2. What further investigation and treatment would you plan?
3. What non-medical advice would you give him?

Case 19

1. The pleural fluid was an exudate containing 40 g protein/l, but there were no pus cells except a few atypical-looking mesothelial cells. The pleural biopsy shows a sarcomatous type of mesothelioma with spindle-shaped cells having abnormal nuclei. The diagnosis is therefore malignant mesothelioma, which in most cases is consequent upon asbestos exposure many years previously. The patient had worked in the shipyards as a carpenter, which meant that he had both sawn and drilled asbestos-containing boards (mostly white chrysotile) used as partitioning between cabins, and had often been working in the immediate vicinity of laggers applying asbestos lagging (which often included blue crocidolite) inside the ships, without any respiratory protection. Later, in his work for the council, he had fitted insulation in houses around the heating systems, and until about 1970 these panels also contained brown (amosite) asbestos. The lance-like fibres of blue and brown asbestos are much more likely to have caused the mesothelioma than the serpiginous white asbestos (**5**).

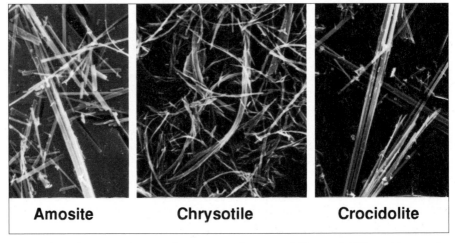

Amosite   **Chrysotile**   **Crocidolite**

5 Scanning electron micrographs contrast the curved fibres of different types of asbestos fibres. (Reprinted with permission from Roggli, Greenberg and Pratt, *Pathology of Asbestos-Related Diseases,* Little, Brown and Company.)

2. There is no curative treatment of mesothelioma, but the average time from diagnosis to death is just over 12 months. It is therefore worth carefully planning palliative care, which means anticipating likely problems. First, his effusion is likely to recur, producing severe breathlessness again. Further aspiration, together with a chemical pleurodesis to occlude the pleural space and thus prevent further accumulation, is well worthwhile. Pain is often a feature, and can be severe. Patients and their carers need to know that if such pain occurs there is help available, either with sustained-release morphine preparations or with specific nerve-blocks or other procedures from a specialist pain clinic. If breathlessness and pain are adequately relieved, the patient's quality of life may be quite good. A CT scan (6) is often performed to delineate the extent of the disease, and this may help in planning treatment. The CT scan is an effective tool with which to display the anatomy, as it can be seen by comparing the scan with the postmortem macroscopic appearances (7) which show how the mesothelioma spreads along the tissue planes to encase, disable and eventually replace the lung within the hemithorax. Lastly, most men who have worked with asbestos are only too aware of the implications of the diagnosis because they will know of colleagues who have had similar problems. Gentle but supportive counselling of patients and family, giving honest but caring answers, can help to ease some of the psychological pressures of the diagnosis.

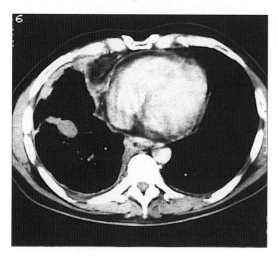

6 CT scan showing the small right lung encased by tumour.

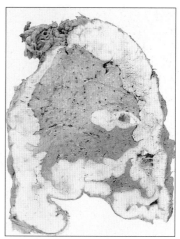

7 Postmortem specimen showing macroscopic appearances.

3. The non-medical advice consists of:

(1) Advising him to put a claim in, via the social security office or his trade union, to the Medical Boarding Centre (respiratory diseases) or other government compensation scheme who will expedite a pneumoconiosis pension in such cases; and

(2) Advising him to discuss his case with a solicitor, since there will often be additional compensation via the civil courts. Although the civil action is rarely completed before the plaintiff's death, it may be comforting to know that dependents are not being left destitute.

Case 20

An unresponsive case

A 62-year-old man presented with a two-week history of flu-like illness with cough, haemoptysis and mild temperature. He had smoked 20 cigarettes a day since he was a teenager, but had stopped a month previously. For some months he had been generally unwell, with intermittent green sputum (but no haemoptysis), and had had difficulty keeping warm. On examination he appeared thin, but there were no palpable glands and no abnormal physical findings in the cardiovascular system or abdomen. His weight was 54.5 kg. A chest radiograph (**1**) is shown; there was some dullness to percussion and bronchial breath sounds at the extreme right apex, corresponding with the abnormality. A CT scan was performed, and cuts through the lesion are shown in **2** and **3**.

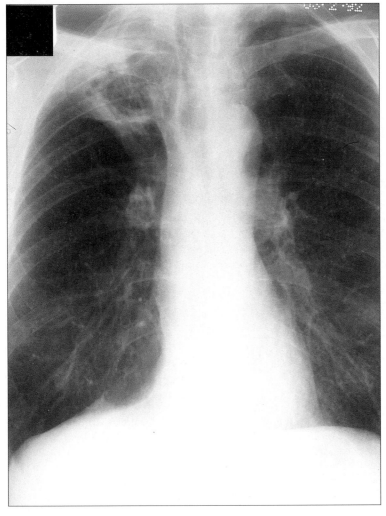

1 PA chest radiograph.

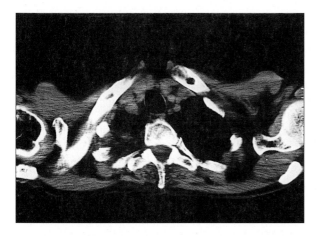

2 A CT scan at level of cavity (mediastinal setting).

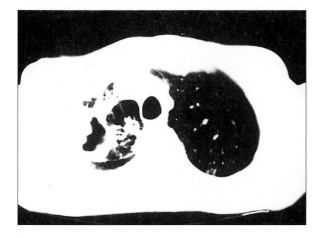

3 The same cut at lung tissue settings.

Investigations

- Bronchoscopy with washings for microbiology, smear and cultures, including examination for acid- and alcohol-fast bacilli

- CT scan

QUESTIONS

1. What is the differential diagnosis?
2. What might the lavage show, and how would you proceed?
3. If cancer were excluded, and there was no response to conventional anti-tuberculous therapy, what else would you consider?

Case 20

ANSWERS

1. There is a cavitating lesion at the right lung apex with collapse/consolidation of the right upper lobe. The most likely diagnosis in a smoker is cancer, but tuberculosis cannot be excluded radiographically. An acute cavitating bacterial pneumonia is unlikely because the man is not ill enough.
2. The bronchoscopy lavage fluid contained cells suggestive of malignancy. Initial washings showed no pathogens on direct smear or culture.

    The patient had no treatment, and six months later a second bronchoscopy again showed no tumour or any organisms on direct smear of lavage fluid, but at six weeks, atypical AAFB were cultured. He was started on tablets comprising a mixture of rifampicin, isoniazid and pyrazinamide.
3. Atypical mycobacteria have very different growth characteristics in the laboratory (4–9). Subsequent identification of the mycobacterium showed it to be *Mycobacterium malmoense* resistant to isoniazid and rifampicin, with borderline resistance to ethambutol but sensitive to ethionamide, cycloserine, clarithromycin and clofazimine. Medication was changed to rifampicin, ethambutol and ciprofloxacin. The patient's initial progress was satisfactory, and his weight improved to 68 kg. Four months after starting medication he felt nauseous, and the medication had to be stopped. Two weeks later he was recommenced on rifampicin and ethambutol, but developed severe skin reactions with abdominal pain and generalised erythematous rash.

4–9 Mycobacteria incubating on Löentgen–Genstein slopes.

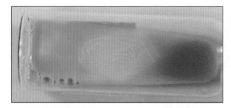

4 *M. malmoense.*

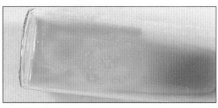

5 *M. kansasii.*

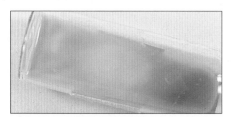

6 *M. avium-intracellulare.*

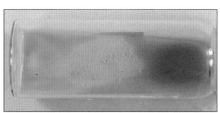

7 *M. tuberculosis.*

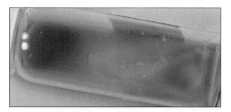

8 *M.marinum.*

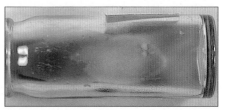

9 *M. cheloniae.*

All therapy was stopped and he was observed on a monthly basis. A month later he was feeling reasonably well, but was having slight pyrexias. After a further month (18 months in total after his initial presentation), he complained of a bad cough production of white phlegm, and that he was feeling generally unwell. His weight had not changed. His chest radiograph showed some improvement in the right apex, but a 5 cm cavity remained. He was referred for thoracic surgery, and a right upper lobectomy was carried out. Afterwards, his operation results showed good progress, with no continuing infiltration in the right apical area (**10**). He stopped all medication and was finally reviewed to be discharged in April 1994, 10 months after his operation. His weight remained stable, he was asymptomatic and was generally well. Cultures of the excised lobe showed no mycobacteria to be present.

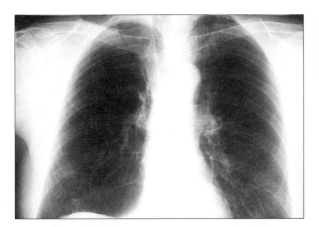

10 PA chest radiograph three months after operation to remove the right upper lobe.

Comments

This man's initial presentation of a right apical pneumonia with cavitation was suggestive of pulmonary tuberculosis. Cultures eventually showed this to be *M. malmoense*, an environmental mycobacterium which rarely causes serious lung disease except in the elderly, those with pre-existing lung disease such as chronic bronchitis or bronchiectasis, and immunocompromised individuals. Specific chemotherapy for these organisms is difficult, as they are resistant to first-line drugs, and second-line drugs frequently cause adverse reactions which make continuous chemotherapy difficult. This individual had reactions to ethambutol and rifampicin, commonly used first-line drugs in the treatment of environmental mycobacterial infections. It was therefore decided that if the lesion could be removed this would provide the best means of cure. In the event, this proved a satisfactory outcome.

Case 21
A wheezy dock labourer

A Liverpool man of 61 years went to see his doctor complaining of increasing breathlessness on exertion 'all the time'. This man had been bothered by several episodes each year of bronchial infection with purulent sputum and acute dyspnoea. He is able to walk the 100 yards slowly to the pub at lunchtime, but is unable to help his wife carry shopping or to do any jobs about the house. He has to stop for breath halfway on a single flight of stairs, and is breathless when dressing and washing. However, once in bed he sleeps soundly, but notices his chestiness immediately upon rising in the morning. He continues to smoke 20 cigarettes each day and has no intention of stopping, as he does not believe cigarettes have played a part in his present condition. Instead he blames his 30 years of work as a welder in the ship-building and ship-repairing yards, and hopes that you will support his claim for compensation. His father died of lung cancer, but there is no other family history of chest disorders. He has two large dogs at home. He was treated for 'anxiety neurosis' in his 40s, and 10 years earlier had a vagotomy and pyloroplasty for a duodenal ulcer. This operation was very successful, and there has been no further stomach trouble. His current medication consists of salbutamol, terbutaline and beclomethasone inhalers (although he finds that none of these are 'much good'), slow-release theophylline tablets and lorazepam to ensure a good night's sleep.

On examination, the patient was comfortable at rest, but was obviously dyspnoeic while undressing. He was pink and had no finger clubbing or signs of heart failure. There were reduced breath sounds over his right lung, and a prolonged expiratory wheeze. There were no lung crepitations and no other positive physical signs. His chest radiographs in inspiration and expiration are shown in **1** and **2**. An ECG showed a mild right axis deviation with some 't' wave changes , but no p pulmonale (**3**). His full lung-function tests are shown in **Investigations**, and CT scans of the lower zones of the lungs in both inspiration and expiration are seen in **4** and **5**. A ventilation perfusion scan was also performed.

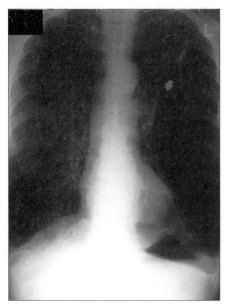 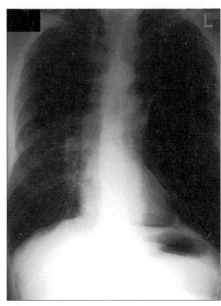

1 Inspiratory PA chest radiograph.   **2** Expiratory PA chest radiograph.

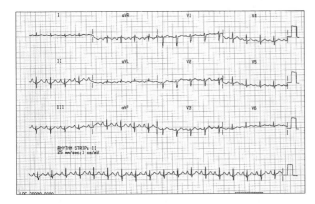

3 ECG.

Investigations

FEV$_1$:	0.55 L	2.7 L
FEV$_1$ post-salbutamol:	0.65 L	
FVC:	1.4 L	3.8 L
RV (helium dilution):	4.3 L	2.2 L
RV (plethysmograph):	5.5 L	
TLC (plethysmograph):	6.9 L	6.1 L
TLC (helium):	5.7 L	
D$_L$co:	15.9 ml/min/mmHg	24.5 ml/min/mmHg

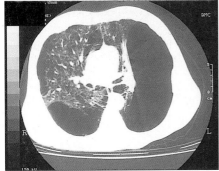

4 CT scan in inspiration.

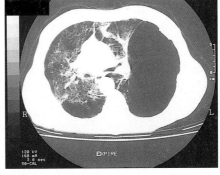

5 CT scan in expiration.

QUESTIONS

1. What is the diagnosis? Has his job played a part?
2. What are the important changes seen on the paired radiographs (**1** and **2**) and CT scans (**4** and **5**)?
3. What blood test might you do, and why would you expect it to be normal in this case?
4. What do the lung function tests show, and what extra information do you still require to plan a treatment strategy for this man?
5. What is the first advice you would give him?

Case 21

ANSWERS

1. The diagnosis is emphysema, which is usually the result of cigarette smoking. His occupation is unlikely to be the cause of bullous emphysema. Welders in the shipyards were exposed to copious irritant fumes, especially when working inside tanks and within the double hulls of submarines. Some developed an acute illness—welding fever fume—at the time, but the evidence is that the fume exposure caused significant long-term damage to the lungs is still lacking. [The ventilation-perfusion lung scan (**5**) shows that there is virtually no ventilation or perfusion to the bullous area.]

2. The radiographs and CT scans show that he has marked bilateral bullous emphysema, which is best seen on the CT scan. There is a huge bulla on the right, and the remainder of that lung has 'collapsed' into a small area medially in the lower part of the chest. On the CT scan the bulla, devoid of any lung markings, is clearly seen on the right, and on the left there is a smaller bulla not immediately apparent from the plain radiographs. The paired inspiratory and expiratory films show that the large bulla is hardly ventilating at all. It remains much the same size in both phases of respiration, and 'pushes' the mediastinum over in expiration as the left lung empties. The bulla is thus acting as a space-occupying lesion within the chest, reducing the volume of lung available for breathing. This is demonstrated well on the CT scan by the contrasting behaviour of the right- and left-sided bullae.

3. When there is extensive emphysema, the possibility of alpha-1 anti-trypsin deficiency should be considered. In this case, the value was expected to be (and was) normal, since smoking patients with this inherited gene defect usually present with lower-zone symptomatic emphysema in their early 40s.

4. The lung function tests show a marked obstructive pattern with an elevated residual volume. The residual volume measured with the body plethysmograph is much higher than that measured by the helium dilution technique, because the helium gas is unable to diffuse into non-ventilated bullae and thus cannot measure the bulla volume. The airflow obstruction is unresponsive to nebulised bronchodilators, in keeping with the mechanical problem in his chest.

   There are two treatment options for this man. Either he could be treated as any patient with COPD, with bronchodilators for limited short-term symptom relief and possibly inhaled steroids if he is steroid-responsive, keeping domiciliary oxygen in reserve if he is hypoxic. Or, he might be considered for surgical resection of the bulla—an operation which, by removing the space-occupying lesion, allows the remaining lung to re-expand and function once again. In carefully selected cases, this major operation can be performed even in elderly subjects with very poor lung function. The most useful extra information required can be obtained by asking the following questions:

   A) Can simple medical measures improve him sufficiently to remove the need for surgical intervention?

   B) Is the arterial $PaCO_2$ raised? (Hypercapnia increases the risks of surgery substantially.)

   C) Is the patient prepared to have major surgery? Some elderly patients will not consider surgery at all.

5. Whatever is to be planned, the first advice should be to stop smoking, as continued smoking is likely to lead to further deterioration and to reduce the chances of successful surgery or successful medical treatment. Simple advice may not be sufficient for such patients, and aids such as nicotine patches (**6**) and counselling are worth trying. This man did stop smoking, and had a number of favourable features for surgery (huge bullae, normocapnia, severe obstruction and evidence of air trapping). Following surgery he was functionally much improved, with an FEV_1 that rose to 1.3 L, and he was able to resume his post as secretary of the local working man's club. His post-operative radiograph is shown in **7**, demonstrating the re-expansion of the residual right lung.

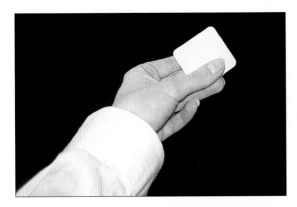

6 Nicotine-containing patch to be placed on the patient's skin.

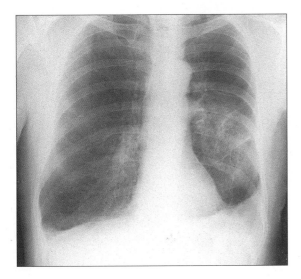

7 Post-surgery radiograph.

Case 22
A chronic productive cough

A 66-year-old lady was referred by her general practitioner with a five-year history of recurrent respiratory infections. Over the past 12 months her symptoms had deteriorated, and she was experiencing approximately one infection every six weeks. She had a chronic productive cough, and during infections produced up to a cup full of purulent sputum per day. Other symptoms included mild wheezing, effort dyspnoea after walking approximately half a mile on level ground, and a recent weight loss of 10 kg. Her only other past illness was a myocardial infarction, and following this she had complained of occasional episodes of angina, which was successfully treated with atenolol. She was a life-long non-smoker.

On examination she looked well; there was no lymphadenopathy or finger clubbing. Examination of the chest revealed mid-to-late inspiratory crackles heard at the left lung base posteriorly, also mild wheezing.

Investigations

Hb:	16 g/dl
WBC:	8.7×10^9/L
Sputum cytology:	Leucocytes +++
Sputum culture:	*Haemophilus parainfluenzae*
Serum proteins:	Total: 58 g/L
	Albumin: 38 g/L
Radiology:	Chest radiograph (**1**)
	High-resolution CT scan of
	lower lobes (**2**)
Protein electrophoresis:	(*see* **3** and **4**)
Aspergillus preciptins:	Negative

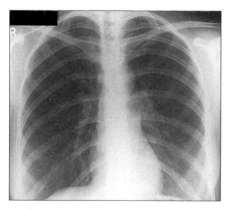

1 Chest radiograph.

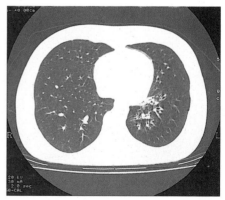

2 CT scan of lower lobes.

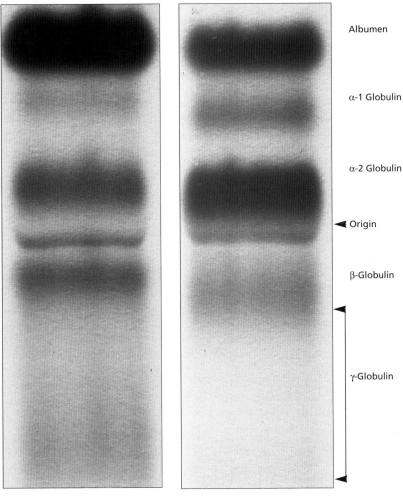

3 Protein electrophoresis, normal.

4 Protein electrophoresis, patient.

Labels: Albumen, α-1 Globulin, α-2 Globulin, Origin, β-Globulin, γ-Globulin

QUESTIONS

1. What is the most likely diagnosis from the clinical history?
2. What do the plain chest radiograph and CT scan show, and what other radiological investigations could be used to confirm these findings?
3. What is the likely underlying cause of this patient's illness, and how would you confirm this?
4. How would you classify these conditions?
5. What general and specific treatments would you instigate?

Case 22

ANSWERS

1. The history of up to a cupful of sputum a day, together with recurrent infective episodes, is highly suggestive of bronchiectasis. The quantity of sputum and the fact that this patient had never smoked makes a diagnosis of chronic bronchitis unlikely. Wheezing is not uncommon in bronchiectasis (occasionally this is associated with bronchopulmonary aspergillosis, but in this case aspergillus precipitins were negative).

2. The plain radiograph (**1**) shows a little shadowing at the left base, which could easily be overlooked. However, the high-resolution CT scans reveal dilated and thickened bronchi, confirming the diagnosis of bronchiectasis. The traditional radiological investigation for bronchiectasis is a bronchogram, which outlines the bronchial walls by instilling contrast medium into the bronchial tree. However, when the CT changes are as clear-cut as in this case, bronchograms are unnecessary.

3. This patient's symptoms have only been present for five years, and there was no preceding severe infective episode. Thus, congenital or post-pneumonic causes are unlikely. In contrast to the usual finding of increased gammaglobulin levels in bronchiectasis, this patient showed reduction in the gammaglobulin fraction. This is highly suggestive of hypogammaglobulinaemia, a rare but well-described cause of bronchiectasis presenting in adult life. The results of the immuno-globulin assays are seen in **Table 1**, and shows a reduced IgM and total IgG, the sub-classes involved being mainly IgG_1. The protein electrophoresis seen in **3** and **4** is from a similar but more severe case, and shows very marked reduction in the gammaglobulin fraction, which is easily seen in comparison with the 'normal' electrophoretic strip.

Table 1   Immunoglobulin results

	Patient value	Normal range
Total protein:	58 g/L	(60–80)
Albumin:	38 g/L	(36–50)
IgG:	4.9 g/L	(6.4–15)
IgA:	1.6 g/L	(0.7–3.2)
IgM:	0.5 g/L	(0.6–2.8)
IgG_1:	2.2 g/L	(4.2–12.9)
IgG_2:	2.1 g/L	(1.2–7.8)
IgG_3:	0.44 g/L	(0.4–1.29)
IgG_4:	0.14 g/L	(0.01–2.9)

4. Hypogammaglobulinaemia associated with bronchiectasis is classified into primary and secondary deficiencies. Primary immunodeficiency may be either congenital, as with X-linked hypogammaglobulinaemia, or acquired, which normally affects adults and is thought to be caused by viral infections. In such cases, it is common for only certain immunoglobulin sub-classes to be affected. Secondary causes of hypogammaglobulinaemia are usually associated with malignancies of the lymphoid system.

5. The general management of these patients is:

A. to treat infective exacerbations with antibiotics, the normal organisms associated with IgG sub-class deficiencies (especially sub-class 2) are poly-saccharide capsular bacteria (*Streptococcus pneumoniae* and *Haemophilus* spp.).

B. Regular daily postural drainage is an important and effective way of reducing the frequency of infections. In this case, the beta-blocking drug was stopped as it is contraindicated in any patient who has airflow obstruction.

C. Specific treatment of the immunoglobulin deficiency can now be achieved with regular replacement of human immunoglobulins (however, IgA deficiency cannot be treated in this way). The current recommendation is for regular intravenous infusion of immunoglobulin, in this case every three weeks. This is carried out slowly with an infusion pump (**5**), as too-rapid administration is associated with the clinical picture of anaphylaxis.

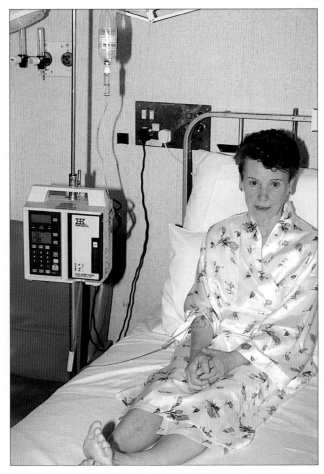

5 Patient receiving intravenous infusion of immuno-globulin through an infusion pump.

Case 23
Years of wheeze

A man of 55 years who smokes 20 cigarettes a day presents to the clinic with a history of breathlessness and wheezing that has been present for many years. Three weeks previously he had developed a cold which went on to his chest, and turned his sputum (which was usually a grey-white colour) green (**1**). His sputum did not clear, despite a course of ampicillin from his general practitioner.

On further questioning, the patient said that as a child he had experienced wheezy bronchitis which had cleared up, and during his teens he had played active sport, including competitive cross-country running. Chestiness had reappeared in his 30s, but until recently it had not interfered with his ability to work or to enjoy family life. He was used to his cough, which was worse in the mornings, and had assumed that it was because he smoked. In the past he had been prescribed two inhalers (one blue and one brown) by his general practitioner, and had taken them regularly for some months. He stopped them because they seemed to be of little value. If he got a cold, his chest was always bad for a couple of weeks (particularly at night), but antibiotics from his general practitioner had always sufficed until this time.

He was married with three children and six grandchildren, one of whom had been diagnosed as an asthmatic. He had a pet cat, but no birds. He worked as a personnel manager for a haulage firm, but was insistent that he never left the office and had no fume or dust exposure. His wife was insistent that the cigarettes were the problem. On examination he was not cyanosed, and was not breathless at rest. He was normotensive and showed no abnormal cardiac or respiratory signs. His ECG and chest radiograph were normal. He performed a spirometry on a wedge spirometer, producing the traces shown (**2**).

The doctor looked at these traces and asked the man to demonstrate how he had been using the inhaler (**3**). He wrote a prescription for two weeks of oral prednisolone and other medication, and arranged to review him thereafter.

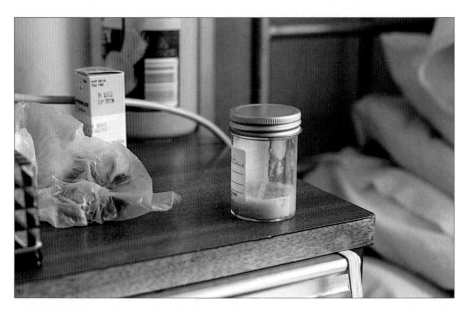

1 Greenish-yellow sputum in a clear pot.

96

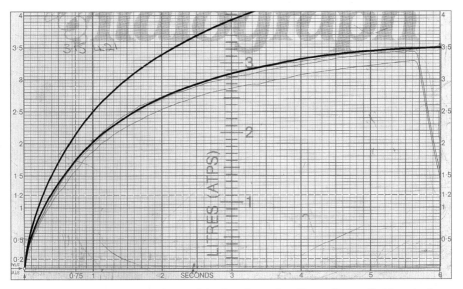

2 Vitalograph and tracings (actual) before bronchodilator (lower line) and after bronchodilator (upper line).

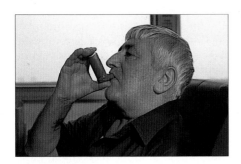

3 Poor inhaler technique (patient was exhaling instead of inhaling).

QUESTIONS

1. Has this man got asthma, COPD or neither?
2. What was the intent behind the steroid prescription?
3. What other medication would you have given him at this time?
4. Which of the many products shown below (**4**) would you consider for him, and in what order?

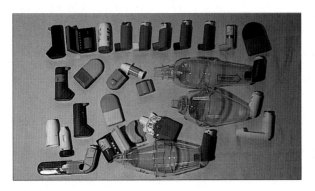

4 Array of inhalers.

Case 23

1. In a smoker aged 55 this is a common clinical problem. There is a considerable symptom overlap between asthma and COPD, and it is not unusual for the two conditions to coexist. This man has a long history of poor response to inhalers, which could suggest COPD, as could the presence of purulent sputum and his heavy smoking history. On the other hand, his spirometry shows that he has an FEV_1 of 1.8 L and an FVC of 3.4 L at rest, yielding an FEV_1/FVC ratio of 53%. (i.e. only mild obstruction of expiratory airflow), which is much improved after a beta-agonist drug as the FEV_1 rises to 2.5 L. This is just above the lower end of the normal range (predicted + 20%) and 38 % better than the resting value. This degree of improvement strongly suggests that he has asthma, but if so, why did he not respond to the inhalers prescribed by his general practitioner? One explanation is shown in the illustration of him taking the inhaler (**3**). The fine particle mist was escaping from his mouth and not being inhaled. Poor inhaler technique is found in up to half of all patients who are prescribed inhalers, and one of the more common problems is to press the actuator after breathing in, so that, although the patient is aware of some particles hitting the back of the throat, most of the smaller particles that could have reached the small airways are exhaled when the patient breathes out.

   Other conditions which have to be considered are bronchiectasis, heart failure and the development of a tumour in the main airways.

2. The doctor prescribed a high dose of oral steroid for just two weeks. Steroids reduce the inflammation in the airways, and thus treat the asthmatic component of the airway disease. By inference, any airflow obstruction not relieved by the steroids is likely to be due to chronic damage from COPD. This is a considerable simplification of the problem, but a trial of oral steroids does seem to be a useful clinical way forward in assessing such patients. In this man, the marked response to beta-agonist and the relatively preserved level of FEV_1 strongly suggests that asthma is more likely, but often there is still value in an oral steroid trial to try and define target levels of PEF against which to assess future treatment. Other tests can be used to differentiate between asthma and COPD (e.g. the diffusing capacity for carbon monoxide or the eosinophil level in the blood), but none are reliable discriminators, and unlike the oral steroid trial, none relate to outcome. After two weeks this man's pre-bronchodilator FEV_1 had risen to 2.4 L and the FVC to 3.7 L. His afternoon PEF values had improved from a range of 240–260 L/min to values of 350–370 L/min, and afterwards he felt better than he had for many years. This makes it almost certain that the primary problem is asthma.

3. This man presented with purulent-looking sputum that had not responded to antibiotics. In asthma the sputum may look purulent because of a high eosinophil content, and therefore the only way to be certain of infection is to culture the sputum. In a man who is not acutely ill and who has a clear chest radiograph, there is no indication for immediate antibiotics. In this case, the sputum was reported to contain *Haemophilus influenzae*, and the patient was contacted at home to arrange antibiotics. He replied that the sputum was already much improved on the steroids and declined the offer.

   He was also prescribed beta-agonist and steroid inhalers as well as a peak-flow meter with which to monitor the response. In addition, an asthma specialist nurse instructed the patient about how and when to use the inhalers and the peak-flow meter.

4. There is a bewildering array of pharmaceutical products available to treat asthma (**5–12**), and British and international guidelines have been established to help the physician make logical choices. There are two components to be considered in such decisions, as follows:

    A) Which drugs?

    B) From which device?

In **5–12**, the various devices are pictured, with some comments about their place in the management of asthma.

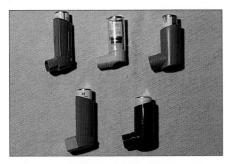

5 Metered dose inhalers (MDIs): cheapest, convenient to carry around, but easy to use wrongly.

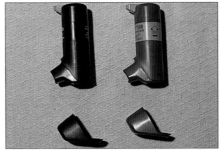

6 Pressure-activated MDIs: more expensive, but still portable and less easy for patients to use wrongly.

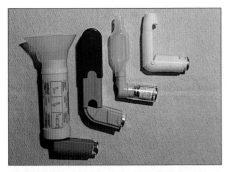

7 Small spacers: more expensive than simple MDIs; more portable, but less effective than large-volume spacers.

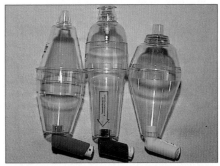

8 Large-volume spacers: cumbersome to carry around, but easy to use. Deliver more drug to airways and less oral deposition. Strongly recommended for use with high-dose inhaled steroids.

Case 23

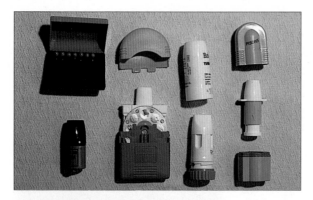

9 Dry powder inhalers: freon-free and preferred by some patients. Less patient error than with MDIs, but more expensive.

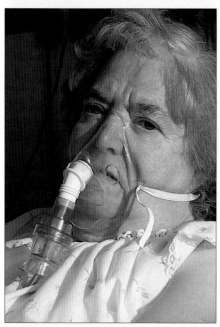

10 Nebulisers: these involve high-dose inhaled therapy, and so are good for acute exacerbations in hospital, but the long-term value is unproven and the treatment is VERY expensive.

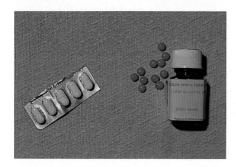

11 Tablets: useful for oral steroids and long-acting bronchodilators. Drugs treat the whole body, not the airways selectively as do inhalers.

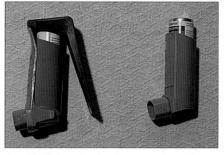

12 Haleraid: for use in patients with arthritic hands.

Case 24
Multisystem disease

A previously fit and healthy 68-year-old woman who was a life-long non-smoker presented with a six-week history of a cough and a feeling of lack of energy. She was initially diagnosed as having a viral illness, but when her symptoms failed to resolve and she started to lose weight she was sent for a chest radiograph (**1**). At this time no abnormal clinical signs were elicited in any system, and the following investigations were carried out:

Investigations

Hb:	10.8 g/dl
WBC:	8.65×10^9 L
ESR:	65 mm in first hour
Urea:	5.6 mmol/L
Electrolytes:	Normal

In view of the above results and the radiograph, a bronchoscopy and transbronchial biopsy was arranged. No endobronchial abnormality was seen at bronchoscopy. A transbronchial biopsy was taken from the right lower lobe. While waiting for further investigations, the patient complained of difficulty with her balance, and her relatives noted that her speech was slurred at times. She developed intense headaches which were most severe in the mornings. Examination showed mild cerebellar ataxia, but no other signs. One of her optic fundi is seen in **2**.

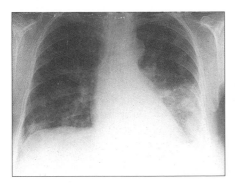

1 Chest radiograph.

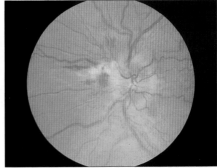

2 Optic fundus.

QUESTIONS
1. Describe the findings on the initial chest radiograph (**1**). What is the likely diagnosis?
2. List the underlying causes of this diagnosis.
3. What other investigations should be performed? Justify your answers.
4. What does the optic fundi (**2**) show? What is the likely diagnosis? What other investigation would you arrange?
5. What treatment(s) would you arrange?

Case 24

1. The chest radiograph shows nodular shadowing throughout both lung fields. The nodules vary in size from 3–10 mm, and none show any cavitation. These appearances are characteristic of pulmonary metastases. The nodules were confirmed on CT scanning of the chest, as seen in **3** and **4**.

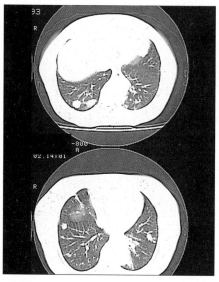

3 CT scan of lower chest.　　　　**4** CT scan of mid-chest.

2. The most common primary tumour sites for pulmonary metastatic adenocarcinoma (**5** and **6**) are the gastrointestinal tract (30%), the genitourinary tract (25%) and the breast (18%). Tumours from the genitourinary tract include renal and renal tract carcinomas, tumours of the testes, prostate, ovaries, cervix and uterus. Other primary tumours are the lung itself, sarcomas, choriocarcinoma, and tumours from the thyroid gland. In up to one quarter of cases (including this case), the metastases may precede the presentation of the primary tumour.

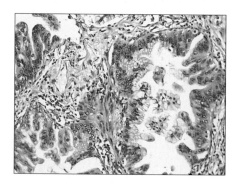
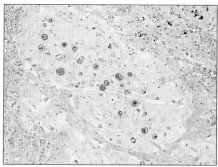

5 Transbronchial biopsy.　　　　**6** Same biopsy, stained for mucin.

3. The further investigations in patients with extensive metastases should be directed at diagnosing the primary tumours which may be responsive to treatment. It is worth excluding a breast neoplasm with a mammogram, as tamoxifen may be beneficial. An ultrasound of the abdomen and pelvis is usually performed, as occasionally surgical treatment of gynaecological primaries is advocated. If there is any suggestion of thyroid swelling, a thyroid scan is indicated, since secondary deposits may respond to radioactive iodine.

4. The optic fundi show the disc margins to be blurred with oedema of the optic cup and surrounding haemorrhages. These findings are characteristic of papilloedema, and are likely to be associated with raised intracranial pressure due to cerebral metastases. The investigation of choice is a CT brain scan, and in this case the CT confirmed multiple tumours in the brain (**7**).

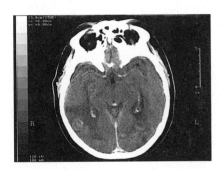

7 CT brain scan.

5. As this patient's tumour was an adenocarcinoma of unknown aetiology, the chance of any benefit from either radiotherapy or chemotherapy is very remote, and the potential side-effects are very severe. In addition, cerebral metastases are very resistant to any treatment. If the tumour was arising from breast, thyroid or embryonic tumours, treatment should be carefully considered. In this case, no specific treatment was given apart from high-dose dexamethasone to relieve the cerebral oedema. However, it is very important that these patients should receive other palliation of their symptoms as these arise, together with counselling and support for both themselves and their families.

Further History

The patient responded well to dexamethasone, but the site of the primary tumour was not found. Two months after commencing steroids, she suddenly deteriorated, experiencing severe unremitting upper abdominal pain which radiated to her back and was associated with severe vomiting. On examination, she was found to have peripheral circulatory failure. Examination of the abdomen showed tenderness and guarding in the epigastrium; the bowel sounds were reduced, but not absent.

QUESTIONS

1. What is the most likely diagnosis, and how would you confirm this?
2. What treatment would you give?

Case 24

ANSWERS

1. This patient had developed an acute abdominal condition associated with peripheral circulatory failure. The fact that she was on steroids raised the possibility of a perforation; however, the bowel sounds were not absent, and the plain abdominal radiograph showed an ileus and no evidence of gas under the diaphragm. The most likely cause for these symptoms is acute pancreatitis, and confirmation of the diagnosis was made when the serum amylase was found to be markedly elevated.

   Acute pancreatitis is usually associated with diseases of the biliary tract, alcoholism, major surgery and a variety of other conditions. Occasionally, it may be the manifestation of a primary tumour in the pancreas, as was the assumption in this case. The patient died within 24 hours of the development of the pancreatitis, and a subsequent postmortem examination confirmed the presence of multiple metastatic disease. There was also a small tumour present in the body of the pancreas, which was subsequently confirmed to be a carcinoma (**8**).

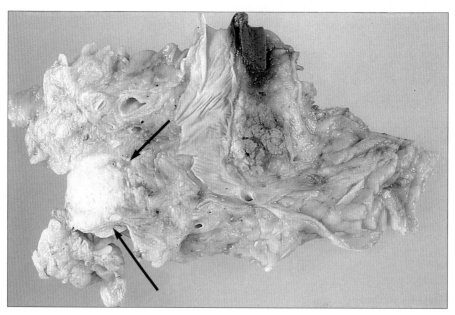

8 Pancreatic carcinoma (*arrowed*) discovered during postmortem examination.

2. Treatment in these circumstances was palliative in view of the underlying diagnosis. Control of the pain was difficult, and required narcotic analgesia. Initially, injections of diamorphine were given. It is well known that continuous infusion of low-dose narcotic analgesia is a very effective way of relieving pain in cancer sufferers, and this was employed with this patient using a syringe driver, enabling her to be pain-free. To control the agitation and nausea, a small dose of haloperidol was added to the diamorphine.

Case 25

Recurrent chest pain

A previously fit 23-year-old man was sitting watching the television when he suddenly developed a sharp, right-sided chest pain, had a bout of coughing and became breathless. His wife noted that he became pale and looked as if he was in severe pain. Within an hour the pain and breathlessness had settled, and he refused to seek medical attention. Over the next two weeks he was a little breathless on exercise, but subsequently all his symptoms disappeared.

Six months later, he had a similar episode of pain while at work and was sent to the local accident and emergency department. When he arrived, the pain was settling and he was no longer breathless. A brief initial examination revealed no abnormal signs; the chest radiograph is seen in **1**. He refused any further tests or treatments and went home. He was back at work within two weeks, but shortly afterwards his symptoms recurred, and he returned to the accident and emergency department. On arrival he was not distressed, and before being seen by the casualty officer an ECG and peak expiratory flow rate (PEFR) were performed (*see* **Investigations**). While the casualty officer was performing the peak-flow manoeuvre, the patient complained of further dyspnoea. Examination of his chest revealed some abnormal signs; a chest radiograph taken at the time is shown in **2**.

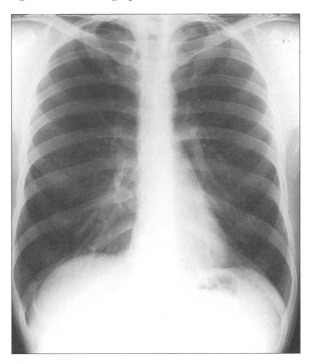

1 Initial chest radiograph.

Investigations

Hb:	14 g/dl	
PEFR:	350 L	
ECG:	Normal	
pH: 7.41	PaCO$_2$: 4.6 kPa	PaO$_2$: 11.2 kPa

Case 25

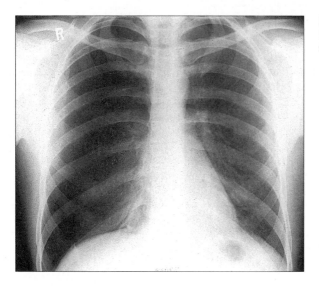

2 Second chest radiograph, revealing some abnormal signs.

QUESTIONS

1. What do the two chest radiographs show, and what abnormal signs were elicited during the chest examination?
2. What treatment would you advise at the time of the first chest radiograph, and at the time of the second chest radiograph?
3. List the causes of the condition you have diagnosed.
4. Should any of the tests not have been requested?
5. Explain in detail how you would undertake any immediate treatment.
6. List the reasons why initial treatment may be unsuccessful.
7. List any complications of the treatment.
8. What treatment should be considered in the future to prevent recurrence of this condition?

ANSWERS

1. The initial chest radiograph showed a small pneumothorax (approximately 20%), which had increased to at least 50% by the time of the second radiograph. There was no evidence on these films of any mediastinal shift, suggesting a tension pneumothorax. The abnormal signs were marked reduction in air entry over the left upper zone, associated with a hyper-resonant percussion note.

2. In the initial radiograph the pneumothorax was small, and thus can be treated conservatively, provided the patient is not dyspnoeic and has ready access to a hospital. If left untreated, a pneumothorax reabsorbs at approximately 1.25% per day. By the time of the second radiograph, the patient required drainage of the pneumothorax with an intercostal tube and drainage via an underwater seal. An alternative is to aspirate air with a cannula and syringe. However, this can only be used if the defect in the pleura has sealed itself. If untreated, the most serious complication is a tension pneumothorax, which may prove fatal.

3. Pneumothorax is divided into two types: primary spontaneous pneumothorax and secondary pneumothoraces due to a variety of chest conditions (**Table 1**). Primary pneumothorax is thought to be caused by a small bulla or bleb at the apex of the lung, and is most common in young men (male to female ratio 3 : 1), and in tall, thin individuals (this patient was 6 feet 3 inches tall).

Table 1   Causes of secondary pneumothorax

- Airflow obstruction (chronic bronchitis, emphysema and asthma)
- Diffuse interstitial pulmonary fibrosis
- Tuberculosis
- Bronchial obstruction (e.g. bronchial neoplasm)
- Cystic fibrosis
- Pulmonary neurofibromatosis
- Lymphangioleiomyomatosis
- Connective tissue disorders (Marfan's and Ehlers–Danlos syndromes)
- Congenital lung cysts

4. It is unwise to perform maximal respiratory manoeuvres in a patient with pneumothorax in case the high transpleural pressures involved produce worsening in the pneumothorax or even precipitate a tension pneumothorax.

5. The immediate treatment is the insertion of a chest drain under local anaesthesia.(**3**). The site of insertion depends on the radiographic findings, but if possible (i.e. in the absence of adhesions) the fifth intercostal space in the axillae is safest (the second interspace in the mid-clavicular line is much nearer vital structures). To prevent lung or tissue damage when the drain is inserted, blunt dissection of the intercostal tissues is carried out. As soon as the drain is in place (**4**), it should be connected to a standard underwater seal. A check radiograph performed afterwards showed that the lung had re-expanded (**5**).

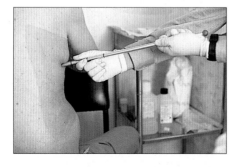

3 Intercostal drainage tube being inserted.

Case 25

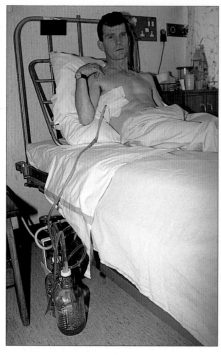

4 Patient with chest drain in place.

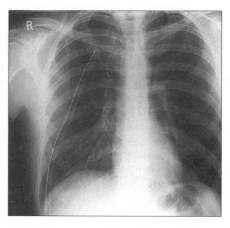

5 Check radiograph performed after draining, showing re-expansion of the lung.

6. If the lung does not re-expand and bubbling continues from the underwater seal bottle, then a low-grade (5–10 cm H_2O negative pressure) high-flow suction can be used by connecting a second bottle specially designed as a 'control valve' (**4** and **6**). If no bubbling is present, check that the tube is patent by observing the water meniscus in the tube is still 'swinging' with respiration.

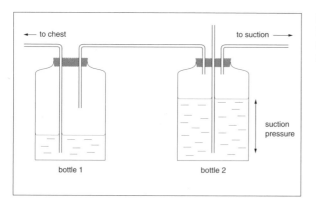

6 Diagram of low-grade high-flow suction using a second bottle as a control valve.

7. The complications of the treatment include damage to various tissues during insertion of the drain, particularly to the intercostal artery, lung or mediastinum. Vaso-vagal shock can occur when passing through the pleura, particularly if local anaesthesia is not optimal. If the tube becomes blocked or is clamped, air may escape around the tube, resulting in surgical emphysema. Alternatively, surgical emphysema can occur due to the escape of air through the mediastinum. A typical radiograph of surgical emphysema is seen in **7**. Bleeding into the pleural space is sometimes seen either spontaneously or due to tissue damage during insertion of the drain. Small pleural effusions are common.

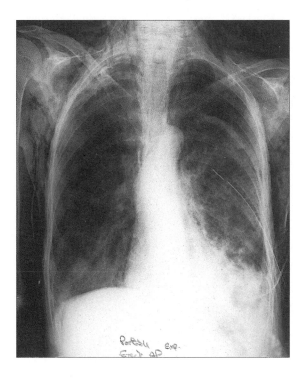

7 Typical radiograph of surgical emphysema.

8. As this patient had recurrent pneumothoraces, surgical treatment was advised. A few months after his admission to hospital he underwent a pleurectomy, and was found to have several bullae in his lung rather than the usual small apical bleb. The apical bullae were removed and the pleurectomy performed. The lung then adhered to the chest wall, making recurrences very unlikely indeed. The diagnosis in this case was congenital bullae, and thus he had a secondary rather than a primary pneumothorax.

Case 26
Hypoxia with normal lung function

A 37-year-old woman presented to her doctor, having coughed up a small amount of bright red blood while walking home from work. She had never been in hospital, and despite smoking 20 cigarettes per day had had no previous cough or phlegm production. However, for the past couple of years she had been aware that she was more breathless than her friends when walking, and she had put this down to her cigarette consumption. Her doctor arranged a chest radiograph (1) and referred her to hospital. At the clinic, the consultant noted a small telangiectatic lesion on her upper lip and that she seemed mildly cyanosed, but examination of the heart and chest seemed normal. The ECG was normal, and spirometry showed normal FEV_1 and FVC at 3.1 and 3.7 L respectively. The haemoglobin was 17.1 g, but she had a packed cell volume (PCV) of 52%. Biochemistry was normal. Her arterial blood gases were measured before and after breathing at 100% oxygen for five minutes.

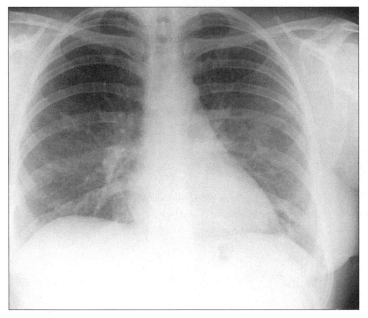

1 The plain chest radiograph which caused the referral to hospital.

Investigations

	On air	On 100% O_2
PaO_2:	6.2 kPa	6.9 kPa
$PaCO_2$:	5.2 kPa	5.1 kPa
pH:	7.41	7.44

A CT scan showed the abnormality quite clearly (2), and this was later confirmed with a pulmonary angiogram (3).

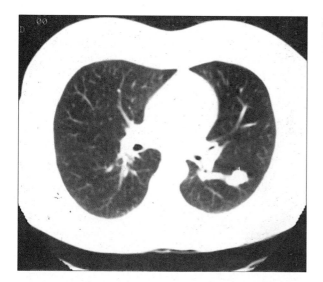

2 CT lung scan demonstrating the lesions seen in **1**.

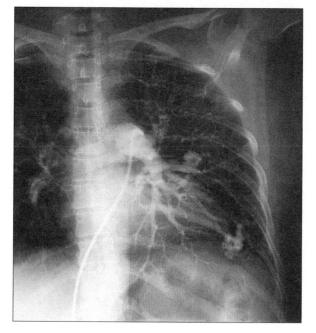

3 A pulmonary angiogram of the left lung.

QUESTIONS

1. What is the diagnosis?
2. Why has the PaO_2 not responded to 100% oxygen?
3. What risks does this patient face in the future?
4. What treatment would you recommend?

Case 26

ANSWERS

1. On close inspection, the plain radiograph shows two smooth shadows in the left lung, which in a smoker with haemoptysis could be due to tumour. However, the CT scan shows that there is a single, prominent feeding vessel supplying the lesion, which strongly suggests that it is a pulmonary arteriovenous malformation. The definitive investigation is angiography, and this revealed that there were not two but three lesions in the left lung, each with feeding vessels. The right lung was entirely normal. Pulmonary arteriovenous malformations occur twice as often in women, and are often not recognised until the third or fourth decade. Haemoptysis and breathlessness are common presenting conditions, but many cases are discovered from radiographs performed for other reasons. About one half of cases have other telangiectatic lesions of the skin or mucous membranes as part of the autosomal-dominant inherited condition Osler–Weber–Rendu syndrome. Whether this lady's single lesion on her lip qualifies as telangiectatic remains speculative—there was no family history to support Osler–Weber–Rendu.

2. The arteriovenous connection causes shunting of blood from the pulmonary artery to the pulmonary veins so that blood does not become oxygenated. This unsaturated blood mixes in the heart with saturated blood from the rest of the pulmonary circulation, and the result is blood of reduced saturation in proportion to the size of the anatomical shunt. Breathing 100% oxygen for 15 minutes has no effect on the blood passing through the malformations, so the unsaturated blood will still be returning to the heart. This prevents a significant rise in the arterial oxygen tension. As a rule of thumb, if a patient remains hypoxic when breathing 100% oxygen, 25% or more of the blood is passing through the arteriovenous shunt.

3. The potential risks are predominantly vascular. Haemoptysis is common but not often severe, although severe bleeding into the lung space can be fatal. The arteriovenous connection may allow systemic venous emboli to reach the brain, and cerebral symptoms are common, although often transitory. Polycythaemia can be severe, with an increased risk of cerebral thrombosis, but patients with Osler–Weber–Rendu syndrome may have bleeding from lesions in the gut or nose and become anaemic. This patient is hypoxic and symptomatic, which usually leads to treatment. In the long term, the shunt size may increase and the hypoxia, symptoms of dyspnoea and fatigue worsen. One iatrogenic hazard is worth remembering: a round shadow on the chest radiograph of a smoker is statistically much more likely to be a tumour than an arteriovenous malformation, and the unwary could be tempted to perform a percutaneous biopsy!

4. This patient is symptomatic and hypoxic, with significant future risks. In the past, surgery was the main option if lesions were in a limited anatomical distribution. Surgery has now been superseded by embolectomy with one of a variety of metal coils, detachable balloons, silicone foams or even 'superglue'. In this lady, the feeding arteries to the three lesions were selectively cannulated one at a time, and a steel coil inserted which thrombosed the feeding artery (4–6). A plain radiograph taken fours years after the procedure shows the metallic coils still in place, and that no new malformations had developed (7). The lady is completely asymptomatic, with an arterial oxygen tension breathing air of 11.2 kPa.

4–6 A longitudinal series of films showing the catheter in place in the feeding vessel.

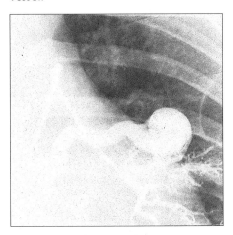

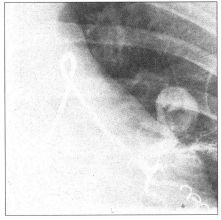

4 Insertion of steel coil.

5 Steel coil in place.

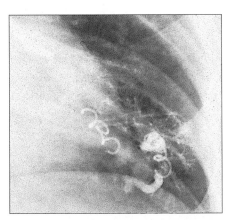

6 Blood supply of malformation ceasing seconds after steel coil in place.

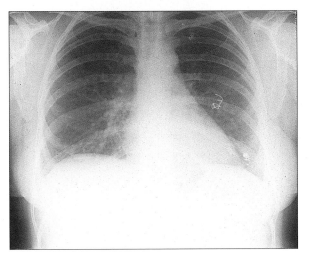

7 Plain chest radiograph four years later.

Case 27
Flushed and breathless

A 59-year-old man who had been feeling 'run down' for about three months noticed that he had lost about 5 kg in weight. He had become a little breathless on climbing one flight of stairs at home, and his chronic productive cough was a little worse than normal. Two weeks before referral to hospital, he had complained of a feeling of fullness in his head, particularly when he bent down, and his wife had told him that his face looked rather flushed. These symptoms slowly got worse, and his general practitioner sent him to the outpatient department. His general appearance is seen in **1**, and a photograph of his upper chest is seen in **2**. In addition, there was an easily heard inspiratory and expiratory musical sound at the mouth. There was no finger clubbing, and examination of his chest revealed both inspiratory and expiratory wheezes. On examination of the abdomen, a smooth liver edge was palpable 2 cm below the costal margin.

The patient was unemployed but had previously worked in the building trade as a labourer on both domestic and industrial sites, including the building of local electricity-generating stations.

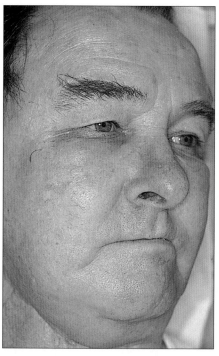

1 Patient's general appearance.

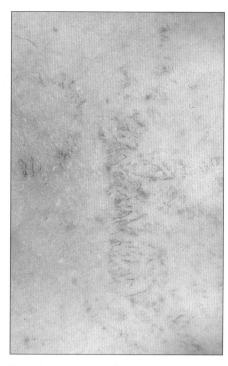

2 Patient's upper chest.

Investigations

Hb:	12.0 g/dl, 10^9/L
ESR:	80 mm in the first hour
Liver function tests:	Normal
FEV_1:	1.2 L (3.4)
FVC:	2.4 L (4.5)
(Predicted values in brackets)	
Flow-volume loop showed attenuation of both inspiratory and expiratory loops with flattened peaks	
ECG:	Normal
Radiology:	Chest radiograph (3)
	Ultrasound of the liver (4)

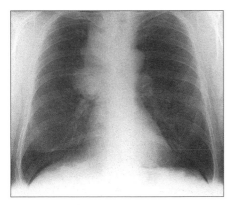

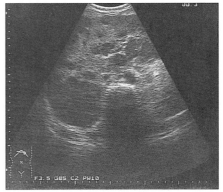

3 Chest radiograph.　　　　　　**4** Ultrasound of patient's liver.

QUESTIONS

1. What do **1** and **2** show?
2. List the causes of this condition, and state what the likely cause is in this patient.
3. What do the wheezing and pulmonary function tests suggest?
4. What does the ultrasound of the liver show?
5. What other investigation should be performed?
6. What treatments are available for the condition shown in **1** and **2**?

Case 27

1. The two clinical photographs show oedema of the head and neck together with a general suffused appearance of the face. The deep and superficial veins were full and non-pulsatile. Over the upper chest were prominent collateral veins, together with some local oedema. These appearances are typical of superior vena caval obstruction. It is common in this condition for the patient to find bending down very uncomfortable, as the blood cannot easily drain from the head and neck. At times the arms and hands can become swollen and painful. A venogram of the superior vena caval system clearly showed blockage at the level of the thoracic inlet, with distal dilatation.

2. By far the most common cause of this condition is a tumour in the superior mediastinum encroaching on the thoracic inlet and compressing the vascular structures (the thoracic inlet is a very restricted space bounded posteriorly by the thoracic vertebrae, laterally by the first rib and anteriorly by the sternum). The chest radiograph confirms a mediastinal mass. Occasionally, compression of the venous system leads to thrombosis of the vena cava and its tributaries. The most common tumour is a right-sided bronchial carcinoma which has metastasised into the paratracheal lymph nodes. This complication occurs in 4% of bronchial carcinomas. Other malignant tumours are also seen, including thymomas and lymphomas, and, very rarely, non-malignant processes such as a retrosternal goitre or granulomatous conditions can cause superior vena caval obstruction.

3. The audible inspiratory and expiratory wheezing associated with spirometric evidence of airflow obstruction and attenuation of both the inspiratory and expiratory parts of the flow-volume loop suggest associated upper airway obstruction, due either to a tumour in the main airway or extrinsic compression of the trachea. It is likely that the inspiratory wheezing was stridor.

4. The ultrasound of the liver (**4**) shows multiple defects typical of metastatic disease. Occasionally, benign cysts in the liver can cause difficulty in diagnosis.

5. The investigation that is needed is a bronchoscopy. Vocal cord oedema may be present, and treatment with intravenous steroids is sometimes advocated. In this man, bronchoscopy showed extrinsic compression of the trachea and main airways, and a biopsy from the bronchial wall is seen in **5**. If diagnosis cannot be obtained by bronchoscopy, mediastinoscopy can usually be carried out safely.

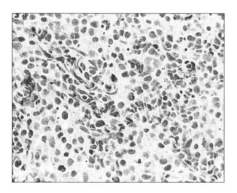

5 Biopsy of bronchial wall showing small-cell lung cancer.

6. It was obvious that there was a malignant cause in this case, and this is most commonly due to a small-cell (oat-cell) carcinoma. The biopsy (5) confirms this, as it shows sheets of small cells with many mitoses characteristic of small-cell carcinoma. Treatments are usually directed to treat the underlying cause. Small-cell carcinoma is often sensitive to chemotherapy, the venous obstruction frequently clearing as a result. Thrice-weekly treatments with etoposide were instituted, and the disease went into remission within four weeks, with complete resolution of the chest radiograph changes. The alternative treatment is radiotherapy. In order to give more rapid relief, a new local technique was also used in this case. A small metal stent was inserted trans-venously into the superior vena cava to allow free drainage until the chemotherapy had had a chance to exert its effect. 6–8 show the metal stent in the superior vena cava. High-dose steroids are often used as an adjunct because of local oedema. Another possible treatment is anticoagulation to control venous thrombosis.

This patient progressed well for eight months, after which his disease recurred and he died of extensive metastatic disease. This sequence of events is very common in small-cell cancers.

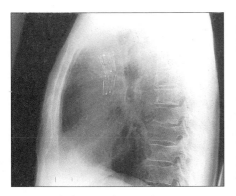

6 Lateral chest radiograph.

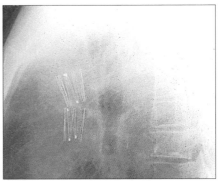

7 Close-up of **6** showing stents in the superior vena cava.

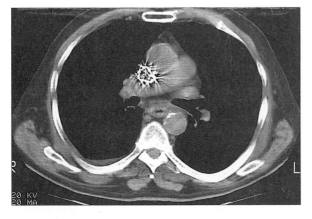

8 CT scan showing metal stent in superior vena cava.

Case 28
A young man in trouble

A 22-year-old male (**1**) was referred by his general practitioner after complaining of a chronic productive cough and exertional breathlessness. However, he had recently moved into the area and no previous medical notes, but he had undergone abdominal surgery in infancy and throughout his childhood had suffered from recurrent chest infections. He had attended a children's hospital until the age of 15, and had left home at the age of 17 years. One of his four siblings had died at the age of 6 years from a respiratory condition. Upon further questioning he admitted to thirst, weight loss and frequent loose bowel motions. On examination he was found to be centrally cyanosed, underweight, of short stature and had marked finger clubbing. His chest was overinflated with an expiratory wheeze, quiet breath sounds, and coarse crackles throughout all areas in both phases of respiration. In the abdomen there was an old mid-line scar, 4 cm firm hepatomegaly, 2 cm splenomegaly, and the caecum was palpable and tender. His chest radiograph is shown in **2**, and his ECG is shown in **3**.

Abdominal ultrasound confirmed the the hepatosplenomegaly, with an echo-bright liver pattern and a dilated portal vein.

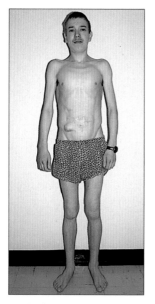

1 Patient on presentation.

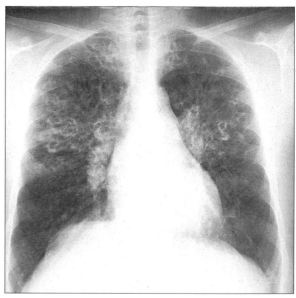

2 Chest radiograph.

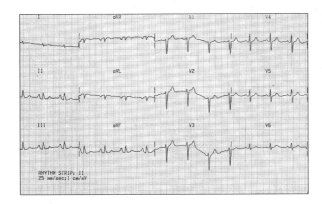

3 ECG.

Investigations

Hb:	16 g/dl	
PCV:	52%	
Spirometry:	PEF:	155 L/min
	FEV$_1$:	0.83 L (4.50)
	FVC:	1.25 L (5.60)
	(Predicted normals in brackets)	
Blood gases:	pH:	7.42
	PaO$_2$:	7.73 kPa
	PaCO$_2$:	4.75 kPa
Biochemistry:	U & E:	Normal
	Sugar:	16 mmol/L
	Amylase:	37 (<200)
Liver function tests (LFTs):	Alkaline phosphatase:	600 IU/L
	Bilirubin:	13 mmol/L
	Alanine transferase	
	(ALT):	65 U/L
Urinalysis:	Protein:	Negative
	Glucose:	++
	Blood:	Negative
Sputum culture:	Profuse *Pseudomonas aeruginosa*	
Faecal fat excretion:	95 g/day	

QUESTIONS

1. What does the chest radiograph show?
2. What does the ECG show?
3. What do the blood gases and spirometry show?
4. What do the abdominal findings show?
5. State the likely diagnosis, and list two possible confirmatory tests.
6. What is the underlying abnormality in this condition?
7. What is the significance of the operation in infancy, and of the history from age 15?
8. How would you treat this patient?

ANSWERS

1. The chest radiograph shows overinflated lungs, with flattening of the diaphragms. There is widespread pulmonary mottling, with bronchial wall thickening and ring shadows, particularly in the upper zones. These changes are typical of advanced bronchiectasis.

2. The ECG shows 'p' pulmonale with right axis deviation. Although these changes can be non-specific, in this case they are due to right heart strain and demonstrate pulmonary hypertension secondary to advanced lung disease.

3. The blood gases demonstrate type 1 respiratory failure, and the spirometry shows marked restriction with airflow obstruction. This pattern is typical of advanced bronchiectasis.

4. Hepatosplenomegaly with a dilated portal vein demonstrates portal hypertension, and the raised alkaline phosphatase with relatively normal hepatic enzymes suggests an extrahepatic cause. The elevated blood glucose and greatly excessive faecal fat excretion are features of gross pancreatic dysfunction.

5. The diagnosis is cystic fibrosis. Confirmatory testing can be performed by means of the sweat test (4) and DNA testing. A universal feature in this condition is an excess of sodium and chloride ions in sweat gland secretions (the sweat test). While this is routinely performed in children, in adults the normal range unfortunately overlaps that of the cystic fibrosis population and the test can therefore be unreliable. DNA testing is absolute, but the defective gene type can only be easily detected in a proportion of patients (86% of Caucasians). Therefore, in a number of patients the diagnosis has to be based on the clinical picture. In this case, the affected sibling demonstrates that the gene defect is inherited as an autosomal-recessive trait.

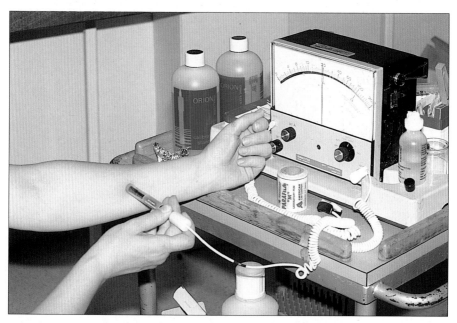

4 Sweat test being performed. The probe heats the underlying skin, causing localised sweating. The electrolyte content of the sweat is then analysed.

6. The underlying abnormality in cystic fibrosis is a failure of cells based at mucosal surfaces to express a transmembrane regulator protein. Although the exact function of this protein is still unclear, it regulates the passage of sodium across the membrane. Secretions at the luminal surfaces thus become dehydrated and sticky, resulting in a failure to clear mucus correctly. In the lungs, this causes chronic infection, bronchiectasis, and progressive respiratory failure. In the pancreas, there is progressive exocrine and endocrine failure. In the gut, there is abnormality of intestinal mucus, and in the biliary system, inspissated bile can cause secondary biliary cirrhosis (as in this man). In the male there is azoospermia due to failure of the vas deferens to develop. In the sweat glands, there is failure to resorb sodium so that excess loss occurs.

7. The operation in infancy was due to meconium ileus, a condition whereby sticky gut mucus (meconium) caused obstruction of the bowel shortly after birth. It is still a major cause of mortality in the first year of life of children born with cystic fibrosis. A similar condition (meconium ileus equivalent) causes bowel obstruction in adults, whereby inspissated mucus collects in the caecum, causing it to become palpable and tender. Many patients with cystic fibrosis, when reaching adolescence, rebel against the strict treatment regimes necessary in this condition and often become lost to follow-up, experiencing subsequent deterioration in their health. This patient's history is therefore typical.

8. Patients with cystic fibrosis require regular daily postural drainage (**5**), pancreatic enzyme supplements and repeated courses of intravenous antibiotics. This patient has already developed respiratory failure, diabetes mellitus and secondary biliary cirrhosis with portal hypertension. He will also require insulin, and should be considered for lung and possibly liver transplantation. He will be infertile and will need appropriate counselling. Although most individuals now reach adult life, the median survival is still less than 30 years. Such patients represent complex medical problems, and are best dealt with at specialist centres.

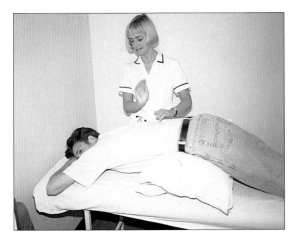

5 Postural drainage being performed.

Case 29

A lady with a shadowy radiograph

A 46-year-old lady went to her family doctor complaining of increasing shortness of breath with ankle swelling and a night-time cough. On further enquiry, she admitted to being aware of breathlessness and a non-productive cough for two or three years. A chest radiograph was reported as showing left heart failure, so she was started on diuretics and referred to hospital. The diuretic did not improve her breathlessness.

She had smoked 20 cigarettes a day for nearly 30 years, but until the last few months had been able to carry on all her household duties and do a part-time job in a wine-merchants. In the last three months she found that she was unable to walk the 800 m to her place of employment or to climb a single flight of stairs without being out of breath. Lifting boxes of wine at work was impossible and made her joints ache; consequently, she had been off work for the past six weeks.

On examination, the jugular venous pulse was not elevated, but there were bilateral fine crackles over the mid and lower zones of both lungs during the second half of inspiration. Her fingers appeared clubbed, but she claimed her fingers (and her mother's) had always been that shape. The liver was not palpable, and there was no ankle oedema. The chest radiograph (1) was unchanged from that of two weeks earlier (before the diuretic). Other investigations showed an elevated ESR of 41 mm in the first hour but a normal blood count and normal biochemistry. A CT scan was performed of the chest, showing abnormalities on both lung (2) and mediastinal (3) windows. Lung function tests (*see* **Investigations**) showed a markedly obstructive picture with no response to nebulised bronchodilators. To make the diagnosis, a further investigation was performed (4 and 5).

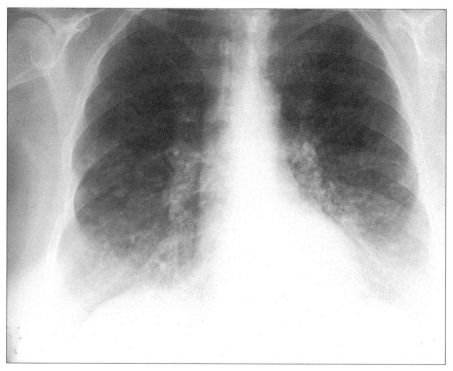

1 Chest radiograph at presentation.

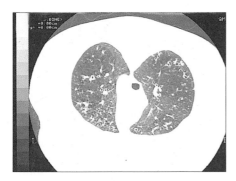

2 CT (lung setting).

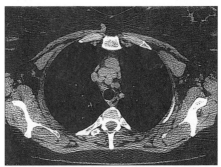

3 CT (mediastinal) setting.

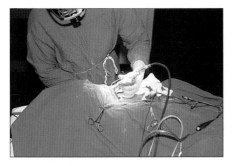

4 Procedure being performed.

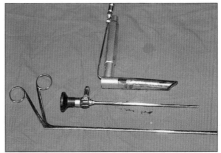

5 Instruments used.

Investigations

	Actual	**Post-nebulised salbutamol**	**Predicted**
FEV$_1$:	0.8 L	0.8 L	2.7 L
FVC:	1.8 L	1.9 L	3.6 L
TLC:	4.5 L		5.4 L
D$_L$co:	24.0 ml/min/mmHg		24.3 ml/min/mmHg

QUESTIONS

1. What are the abnormalities in the chest radiograph and the CT scan?
2. What is the investigation shown in **4** and **5**, and what are the two most likely diagnoses?
3. Why is her long cigarette-smoking history alone insufficient to explain the clinical picture?
4. Her employer writes to you asking if and when this lady will be fit to return to work. How should you reply, and what is her prognosis?

Case 29

1. The chest radiograph shows a diffuse infiltrate throughout both lungs which, because of its distribution, it might be confused with the upper lobe blood diversion of left heart failure. However, there is an additional abnormality in that the hilar glands are significantly enlarged, particularly on the right side where they are clearly demarcated inferiorly and medially. The CT scan (**3**) of the upper chest shows multiple enlarged nodes alongside and in front of the trachea. Other sections confirmed the bilateral hilar nodes, best seen using lung window settings (**2**). There are multiple infiltrates in both lungs which are clustered around the bronchi. These infiltrates were widely distributed, but were maximal in the upper lobes. An important negative finding is the absence on the CT scan of any evidence of emphysema. This makes it less likely that the clinical disability can be explained simply by cigarette-related COPD.

2. The procedure shown in **4** and **5** is a mediastinoscopy (performed using general anaesthesia) in which the surgeon inserts a mediastinoscope into the neck to access and sample the mediastinal lymph nodes. The procedure is most commonly performed as part of the pre-operative assessment of potentially resectable pulmonary tumours in order to exclude secondary spread. In this case, there are two possible causes of the extensive lymphadenopathy: sarcoidosis and, less probably, lymphoma. Histology of the nodes provides the most direct and most certain method of achieving a definitive diagnosis. The histology of the lymph node (**6** and **7**) shows the classical non-caseating sarcoid granulomata with well-marked giant cell formation. A bronchoscopy performed under the same anaesthetic showed reddened and inflamed bronchial mucosa, but no focal stenoses. Bronchial biopsy alone will usually provide histological evidence of sarcoid, but cannot exclude for certain other processes in enlarged lymph nodes. Indirect confirmation of sarcoid comes from the serum angiotensin-converting enzyme level, which was mildly elevated.

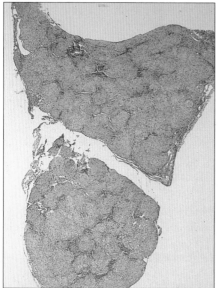

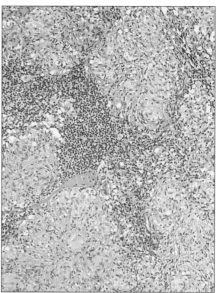

6 Histology (low power) of the lymph node.

7 Histology (high power) showing well-marked giant cell formation.

3. The lung function tests showed a distinct obstructive defect which is sufficient to explain her marked symptoms, and which could be compatible with COPD secondary to her cigarette smoking. Some of her airway obstruction may be due to smoking-related small airways disease, but COPD cannot explain the radiographic shadowing, the lymphadenopathy or the fine crackles on auscultation. Sarcoid can cause an obstructive defect with large airway stenoses or with widespread small airways disease.

4. Assuming you have the patient's permission to reply, then the employer is effectively asking what the prognosis is for sarcoid. In the short-term, the pulmonary infiltrates, lymphadenopathy and breathlessness may respond well to high-dose oral corticosteroids (40 mg/day). This lady felt much better within four weeks; her FEV_1 improved to 1.4 L, and her infiltrates were less marked. The longer-term outlook should be more guarded. Patients with hilar lymphadenopathy alone (with or without erythema nodosum) almost always resolve spontaneously, and have an excellent prognosis. When there is pulmonary shadowing there may be an excellent resolution, or the sarcoid may be healed by fibrosis, leaving a scarred lung that may be susceptible to recurrent infection or to colonisation by *Aspergillus*. The sarcoid may continue to progress in spite of steroid therapy, ending in chronic respiratory failure. **8** is a postmortem lung from another patient who died of progressive sarcoid. The nodular abnormal areas can be seen macroscopically and on histology (**9**). The focal granulomata, interspersed with normal alveoli, are easily seen. Thus, the answer to the employer should be delayed for some weeks after commencing treatment, and while in this case can be reassuring in regard to her immediate employment, it should avoid any long-term predictions.

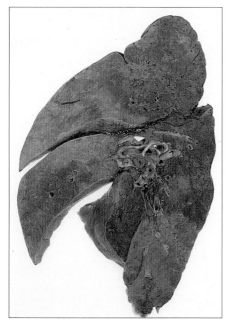

8 Postmortem lung.

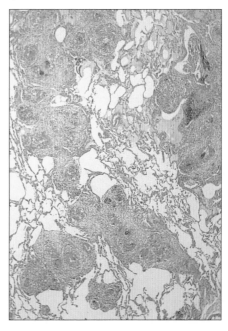

9 Histology of **8**.

Index

Index